Belle Berroyer was born in Essex where she started her professional career in early years development and education. Throughout her varied career, she continued her professional studies, combining both academic research and practical experience knowledge.

In more recent years, she has written articles for various magazines and media platforms, as well as creating and delivering workshops on sensory awareness and autism for early years courses across the academic spectrum, as well as specific workplaces and support services for a multitude of neurotypes, particularly autism.

She has recently set up her own website where she offers environment support for families within their own homes, as well as 1-1 sessions for parents, carers and workplaces to enhance their knowledge of sensory awareness in autism.

In 2002, she relocated to mid-Wales where she became a mother. This is where her awareness of autism and sensory processing became truly active. Her son was born a non-speaking autistic. Teaching her his way of being human, she began to enquire deeply into the sensory aspect of living life. In doing so, she learnt about her own sensory challenges, which answered a lot of before, unknown questions about her own struggles growing up.

Now, 17 years on, Belle has created this practical and insightful introduction to learning the language of autism through the sensory systems.

I dedicate this book to Jerome, my soul mate, friend, husband, mucker and co-parent. My oh my, how I continue to miss you, every day and in every way—as soon as we lay eyes on each other, love arrived.

Thank you for your light, you were uniquely wonderful, you got me just as I am. I always appreciated that—we came into each other's life at the perfect time, creating the wondrous and magnificent Jeorge.

You always believed in my ability to express in words anything I wrote or spoke about autism and sensitivity. Listening to me read aloud my articles, always praising and supporting. Your opinion always mattered—your love cherished by me.

Although, you went far too soon, I wasn't ready to say goodbye to you my darling, 2 years on and look! My book has been written, you are etched in the pages, for I felt you as I wrote each word, encouraging me every step of the way.

I am so glad you heard my soul's call when I asked for you to come into my life. Now our amazing son has grown into a young man—we can continue life here in the physical, knowing and remembering your love remains with us always. We are still co-parenting and will forever remain a family.

I also dedicate this book to Jeorge Berroyer, our beloved son—the brightest light I know. You are my inspiration and teacher, I have learnt through you how to live in the present moment, express yourself without apology and find the pleasure in everything that you choose to do.

You, darling Jeorge, have taught me more about myself than I ever knew I could. I am truly blessed to be your mum and I am grateful every day.

Belle Berroyer

LEARNING THE LANGUAGE OF AUTISM

Through the Senses

AUSTIN MACAULEY PUBLISHERS™

LONDON * CAMBRIDGE * NEW YORK * SHARJAH

A CIP catalogue record for this title is available from the British Library.

ISBN 9781398495128 (Paperback)
ISBN 9781398495135 (ePub e-book)

www.austinmacauley.com

First Published 2023
Austin Macauley Publishers Ltd®
1 Canada Square
Canary Wharf
London
E14 5AA

Writing this book has been a long-time ambition of mine, I know I have at least 3 more sitting in my brain ready to burst out—perhaps there will be more after that.

Throughout my life, I have been blessed and met people who have inspired me in a variety of ways.

One inspirational person I feel I want to highlight is a teacher from when I was in primary school, her name was Angela and she emotionally supported me at a time when I really needed it.

Although at the time I did not realise the impact she would have on me, I have come to realise she was the only one throughout that very challenging time who offered me kindness. She acknowledged my sensitivities and nurtured me. She was gentle in her approach and I felt protected in school because of her awareness of my needs.

She taught me about compassion and the need for a child to feel safe in an overwhelming environment. She gave me what I needed as I stood out from the classroom crowd.

I wish to thank my mum for her love and support over my life, particularly these last few years since the passing of my son's dad—which was so very tragic and overwhelmingly heart-breaking for me. She held me emotionally and has egged me on in her praise and belief that I could get this book finished and published. I love you, Mumma.

My friends are important to me, I cherish them as they come and go through life, each one has reached into my heart and enriched my life and influenced me in one way or another.

I thank you for your company, time shared, adventures had, the laughing until our bellies ached, the dancing, singing and opportunities to expand and grow as a person.

To Carol Cumber, you have inspired me, loved me and helped me see my true self. Through the years, your unconditional love has enriched my life deeply. I cherish you and all that you are darling, I love you.

My soul family, we have shared experiences together that go deep into the soul. We have travelled to beautiful lands and spread our love vibes. Thank you for your continuous love and support for me and Jeorge, particularly these last few years when I have needed it most.

The biggest love in my life is my son, Jeorge, he has and continues to be my greatest teacher. Seeing the world as he does from different perspectives which enables one to recognise the beauty, whether a tree, a flower, piece of material or a sound, his natural self-expression of the environment is captivating—he has taught me to be me, in all my glory. My love for him is boundless, my pride for him is as big as the Universe. The world's perspective he has invited me into has been spectacular—he has enriched my life in every way.

A special acknowledgement goes to Ellie, thanks for consistently probing me about writing my first book and knowing that it was possible, I love you.

During this process, I have needed assistance financially to help get my book published, as an unknown author writing about a complex subject—I was part funded, to which I am truly grateful to my publishers for seeing the potential and believing in my book. I set up a GoFundMe page to help raise the remaining monies so that I could fulfil my financial contract.

As part of my giveback of thanks for donations made, I said I would give acknowledgements individually, so here it goes:

A huge and heartfelt thanks to you all for believing in me and my book, some of you I know personally, some I have never met or spoken to my whole life.

For the anonymous donators, please know you are forever in my heart for your kind contributions in helping me create this book that I am so proud of.

To Uncle Terry and Aunty Sandra, Jayne and Steve (wow)—so very generous—Val and Charles, Liza, Emma, Christine G and Christine C, Darlene, Siwan, Parul, Nia, Tanya, Roger, Cathryn W, Jill, Gill, Lesley, Hannah, Julia, Anne, Jo, Dawn, Rob, Paul, Ashley, Mandy, Susan, Irene, Deborah, Steve, Giselle and Beth, Kath and my dad and step-mum, Helen, Carol and Nick C, Carol W, Stephen, Ruth, Esther, Molly, Catherine and John and Clara.

Table of Contents

1
Disclaimer

The information in this book is by no means meant or intended as a cure for autism in any way. I do not believe or support the idealism that autism should be cured or eradicated.

I am not a medical professional and do not suggest any of the content in this book are cures or will align with every autistic child or adult who ever lives.

This book is intended to create openings to a different way of thinking about what autism is and how an autistic person whatever their age can be supported.

I do not claim to be an expert in matters of autism or that any information in this book is a "one size fits all".

I support that every autistic person is an individual and will each have their own unique methods of communication, their own behaviours, needs and coping strategies.

My use of examples of possibilities throughout this book are by no means exhaustive.

The information in this book has been experienced firstly by my own sensory needs, secondly of my son's and his experiences and communications. Thirdly of a mix of the 100s of autistic people I have met with either physically or through the form of social media.

My intention for this book is to provide sensory information and perspectives so that the autistic person's (child's) life can be supported without the need to be changed or compromised, masked or conditioned to the needs of others, including school, nursery, home, work and life generally.

My intention is to also advocate positively for an autistic child's right to play and have a child hood that is celebrated and enjoyed.

I support the need for a unity approach to supporting a young child's growth and development with outside agencies of teachers, social workers, psychologists, speech and language/communication therapists (S+L) Occupational Therapists (OT), Learning Support Assistants (LSAs) working alongside the child and the parents/carers.

I support the right for an autistic child to be accepted in all areas of their lives, including stimming, their choice of communication whether it be vocal, words, sound, AAC device (communication device) physical, sign, drawing, writing or any other form of communication preferred by that individual and that it is recognised and honoured by others.

I support the right for every autistic child to be given the same opportunities as any other child and in doing so, equally accommodating their needs in order for those opportunities to be attainable to them.

I support the need to ensure you have medically checked that your child is not in any physical pain through any other reason, such as; food allergies/intolerances or other medical conditions unrelated to autism or sensory processing in any way.

Not everything about an autistic child's behaviours is typical of their autism, sometimes their body needs medical attention too. Be sure to not assume it is a typical behaviour of autism and so ignoring what could be a serious medical condition whether it is temporary like a stomach upset or a more serious condition.

Throughout this book, I will use a multi-identification method— meaning I will use a variety of terms such as autistic child, adult and autistic person when speaking of the autistic human. I will use terms such as parent, carer, neuro typical person and professionals. Instead of listing them all in every sentence, I will mix it up throughout to be inclusive. My intention is that throughout the entirety of this book, I am referring to both autistic adult and child as well as any person who is a carer in any capacity to the autistic person, including any professionals who spend time, however small, with the autistic person.

2

Introduction

Firstly, I want to express my deepest gratitude to you for reading these pages. I hope it brings some insights and adds inspiration to your life. Whether you are a parent/carer/family member or a professional who supports an autistic person of any age, whose sensory needs are sensitive in any way.

My intention is that you will feel empowered to stand beside your autistic person advocating for them the best possible environment that enables them to be seen, heard, accepted and honoured exactly as they are.

So here I am offering my wisdom, my viewpoint, my experiences as a mother to a nonspeaking autistic person. I am neurodivergent highly sensitive in areas of auditory, visual and smell as well as being extremely empathic, often feeling the energy of others. My mind can become scrambled when experiencing numerous external sensory inputs. I have an inability to think clearly when presented with too many words on a page, with them often escaping up and out the top of my head.

This has meant that writing this book has proven challenging sometimes—as long as I didn't look up at the typed pages too often, I managed, taking very regular breaks which, I have learnt to do so that I can enjoy the experience of writing, which I absolutely love.

I will share a little background information about me before we delve into the main part topics of the book.

I had enjoyed a varied career for 17 years in early years development and education before I gave birth to my son. I gained a wealth of experience of children's wisdom which I soaked up and stored inside of me. The studying I had completed to get the required qualifications was easily overshadowed by the teachings of the children themselves.

During a job I had as a family support worker, at break time I sat in the staff room, where, on the coffee table, I came across a book titled *The Ultimate Stranger*. At first glance, the cover picture along with the title looked like a thriller novel. I picked it up and began reading.

It was written by a Dr Carl H Delacato, at closer look I discovered this was a book about autism. Dr Carl spoke of sensory over and under stimulation in all areas of the body's senses. It didn't discuss the need to change the child, instead to look and study an autistic person's behaviour through the lens of sensory stimulation. What was the behaviour of the person telling you? Where did they feel overwhelmed and why? Only once this was figured out, changing the environment for them was what was seen and proven (by him) to be of benefit to the children. There was no speak of cures or behavioural training of any kind! This book was seen as revolutionary and stated so across the front page. At that time (1998), I was pretty much in the dark when it came to autism, I had heard the word but that was all. Autistic children were not seen in nurseries, at least not in my experience. (Although I looked back and realised, I had met autistic children, only there was no diagnosis and their label was often negative and derogatory.

I had no idea that in 6 years' time, I would meet my son who was to be a non-speaking, sensory sensitive autistic person. Little did I know this one book (although I did not like the title and still do not) was to be the most useful book I was to read regarding autism.

Jumping forward those 6 years when it became clear (to me) that my son was autistic (he was around 13 months old), I started reading countless books. Sadly, I dived straight into the fear factor, not because he was autistic but because I didn't know what I was doing, how could I support my boy?

The years of being taught by the many children I had cared for and had supported for 17 years seemed of no value to me in my new role as a mother. I had worked in numerous nurseries, primary and social care settings and knew first-hand how unaccommodating and inexperienced most settings were for children with the complex needs my son had, which included myself! We did a tiny section of training under the heading of Special needs, autism back in 1986–88 was not mentioned. For a while, I lost myself, giving away all my power, intuition and self-belief. So heavy was this that I could not see that my son was showing me the way, his way.

I was in a blind ongoing circle of panic and fear, I became irrationally protective of him, seeing him judged and looked upon as odd was too much for my nurturing heart and own sensitivities. When I remember back to that time, I was like a trapped lioness with her cub who I stood in front of so no one could touch or try to change. To me he was perfect, I simply did not know how to support him, worse still my thinking was, how do I stop others from hurting him through their lack of understanding him? If I could not understand or support his needs how on earth was anybody else going to?

Being in a frenzied emotionally charged state of panic, I had forgotten about the book I had read 6 years previously that had filled me with wisdom I did not know I would need (but what my son would need me to know!).

This self-doubt and panic mentality went on for about 2 years, reading as many books on autism as I could hoping that one of them would give me all the answers, I needed to be a better parent. I hoped that somehow, they would unlock some kind of code of understanding autism which would help me understand my son.

After about book number 8, I felt more confused and overwhelmed than I could cope with. I became extremely anxious about his future. I wasn't sleeping properly and my son wasn't getting the mum he deserved. Thankfully, my son's father strongly recommended I stopped reading books as it was, in his words, driving me slightly around the bend!

All I could think of was the future, way, way ahead into the future, it is said somewhere that if we think too much about the past, we become depressed if we think too far into the future, we become anxious. I was doing both, wondering if I had done anything in my pregnancy or before then that could have caused my son to be autistic. Remember I knew nothing about autism and the content of some of the books I was reading at the time were negative and giving incorrect information. This was fuelling a depression and adding anxiety as I worried about his future. (I now know he was born exactly the way he was meant to be, no blame, shame or bad decision by me, before or during my pregnancy.)

So I took his dad's advice and stopped reading the books. Realising I had kept reading because I never found the one that actually gave me the advice, I felt I needed, I wanted inspiration, something to stop me feeling scared and overwhelmed so I could be the parent my son deserved to have.

Once I stopped reading, I remembered all those children I had cared for in previous years and how they had taught me about child development, naturally as they navigated their environment and experienced it. (Not some textbook tick box guideline) I also remembered the book I had read those 6 years previously and how I was innocently fascinated by the words and explanations of these so-called "strangers" that the then world did not understand and would either lock up in mental institutions or strongly advise their parents to do so. Many kids were abandoned by their parents because of the advice of professionals in the field of psychology and Science.

Dr Carls findings with regards to Sensory awareness was the key to many parents seeing their once extremely distressed, self-harming children to becoming happier and non-self-harming by adapting the environment to their individual needs. Rather than change the child.

This changed the lives of these families; they were the lucky ones for at that time (mid 60s) this view was not realised by the masses in professional fields of psychology. Dr Carl was ahead of his time. I was thankful that he helped those he did and so grateful I somehow was guided to read the book myself, which I still have to this day.

In recent years including the present day, there are articles written on various researches into the autism brain that discuss the sensory aspect of the brain being the most pronounced. If you are interested in the science, it is worth researching.

My main point here is that once I took a breath and stopped panicking, I started to think in a more complex manner. I realised that all I needed to do was to listen and by listening, I mean watching and listening with every part of me to what my son was showing me.

As I write these words, there are many actually autistic folks who speak freely to the world about autism. They are advocating for autistic and neurodivergent individuals, supporting neurotypical parents/carers and professionals in the hope that the suffering and misunderstanding that many had experienced in their younger years would be avoided for the generations of today and the future. I hope and it's my intention that this book is seen as a part of that movement.

Chapter 1
So What's This Book About?

I am not a biologist or scientist so this book will be free from using medical and scientific language. There are plenty of websites and books that can be used as research to further investigate and understand what sensory systems our bodies are made up of. This book is written in what I would call everyday language.

I know from personal experience, when I am tired and full of unanswered questions with a dose of worry about the unknown—the last thing I need is a book full of long and complicated medical and scientific terminology that I need a dictionary to translate the meanings of. My aim is that this book is read with ease, when you put it down to do something else, you can later pick up where you left off without having to re-read chapters.

Parenting or caring for a child or adult who has differences of levels of support needs whether medical, physical, emotional, or neurological— emerges you into a world of medical and assessment language. Suddenly new terminologies and phrases are used in meetings and anything you read will have such words that you may have never read or heard of before.

It isn't unusual to be engaging with multiple organisations who all use a particular "professional" language. Unless you are familiar with such language (usually only when you professionally work within those areas) during the numerous assessments processes your child goes through to receive a diagnosis and support this can be overwhelming, confusing and intimidating.

Misunderstandings and frustrations can arise if the language isn't explained so that you can successfully take part in the conversations around the table. Much of the current language used within the diagnostic processes are both terminologically and factually incorrect. (As previously mentioned, such wording used to diagnose are being challenged by Autistic communities with success. New terminologies are being born so that each of us can help create a language that is supported and preferred by the autistic people whom you wish to support and advocate for.)

During this pre/assessment time your child suddenly becomes an array of descriptive and verbal words, a diagnosis, a label, a statistic based on whatever evidence science has up to that point, come up with. Alarmingly some phrases and labels used are in fact not science evidence based but are presented as if they are. This is something to be mindful about.

Currently there are still methods and trainings offered that claim to have scientific evidence that they can "improve or completely eradicate unwanted behaviours". Looked at more closely these methods can be harmful and, in some cases, inhumane to any person subjected to them.

For example, in the 1960s Ivar Lovaas founded applied behavioural analysis (ABA), he felt that autistic children needed to be spanked and given electric shock treatment to stop self-harming behaviours. He saw autistic children as blank slates that could be moulded and re programmed into looking and behaving "normal" (not my words but his) There is a lot of website papers and interviews of him speaking this philosophy of his. Prepare yourself if you choose to research him, much of what he says regarding the punishment theory is ugly reading. Some centres still practise electric shock treatment to autistic people. YES—shockingly it does still exist, in some countries around the world.

As most of us (parents and carers) especially, have no experience in such things we tend to believe the words said to us without question. Feeling at a loss to know how to help a child from self-harming and hurting others, can lead to making decisions that can cause long-term damage to the autistic child. This is a huge debate currently and you will find plenty of information on plans to eradicate ABA along with its practises. You can find a lot of information about this on autistic led social media groups.

There are other ways that can support an autistic child to stop self-harming—I am hoping that this book will provide you with a deep insight into some of them.

Although most people would, in more modern times, feel the practises of Lovaas as inhumane and would never agree to such treatment. However, his philosophy is still being practised within ABA in varying degrees of intensity. It is beneficial to do detailed research at all times when seeking any type of support or therapy for your autistic/ sensory sensitive child.

The term Asperger's for example is now deemed void by the vast majority of the autistic community. (Not all) Some autistic people prefer to identify as Asperger's and that is their prerogative.

However, it has been removed from the diagnosis list in many Countries in recent years, instead Autism is used across the board. The reasons for this are documented in the aforementioned social media groups and other autistic community platforms, as well as online research.

Many other labels are still around and depending on where you live in the world—you will come across variations of terminology that are intended to compartmentalise "levels of autism". Before you realise it, the child has become a functioning label or category type, when prior to them being diagnosed, they were an individual person with support needs.

My intention is that this book and its content will help you to be continually aware of this, regardless of any labelling they are given. We want to be mindful to not let your child/client get lost and hidden behind all the labels and stereotypes.

Please do not misunderstand, I am not speaking of a diagnosis—autism is the diagnosis, it is the labelling I am referring. They can differ depending on what country/state/County/Province you live, here are some examples Level 1, 2, 3 autism or high and low functioning, even moderate and severe autism.

The latter are labels not diagnoses. This is important to remember, although they may seem harmless and may make sense at the time. The problem with them is it tends to create a façade of what the actually autistic person needs, regarding levels of support and where it is needed. By having a label of high functioning autism (it may be given to you as if it is an official diagnosis), remember the autism part is the diagnosis—the high functioning one is not.

The reason these labels are unsupported by autistic people is they can be misleading and unhelpful to the actually autistic person.

Many of us are able to function with ease in certain situations and environments based on many factors. Whilst on other times not so much or at all. For reasons such as personal health, tiredness, environment, previous experiences that day, week or month, even year.

Triggers can be set off from a memory or association of a memory, the list goes on. Therefore, the label of high functioning (HF) is too limiting as well as having an unrealistic expectation of what and how the autistic person behaves and responds and is capable of being, achieving or able to cope within that moment.

The same happens with the Low Functioning (LF) labelled children, many who are not given opportunities that a "high functioning" labelled person would because they are deemed as LF in every aspect of their existence.

Imagine being labelled as a LF person based on a limited insight into your whole personality, being ignored or deemed unable to do A, B or C. The same relates to being labelled HF and everyone expecting you to have higher levels of coping at everything you do or experience, but when you are experiencing overload, executive functioning difficulties (there is a chapter explaining this further along the book) or sensory difficulties, you may be told to stop acting too autistic or stop pretending (for example) purely on someone else's opinion and expectations of what they have because of their understanding or personal interpretation of the HF label.

Autistic children have needs and desires like neurotypical children. Their innocence needs nurturing and protecting so that they too can enjoy their child hood, even if that looks different in every way to their neurotypical peers. Once into adulthood they will look back at their childhood, they deserve to have memories of fun activities and adventures, rather than a childhood that is only full of therapy and stress. Parents deserve to share in those happy memories too.

Time flies by and it would be a great sadness if their childhood was governed by therapy sessions, distress and misunderstandings of their needs and communications because on every report or assessment the labels were incorrect, untrue or demeaning.

I have already briefly mentioned the book I came across called "The ultimate stranger, the autistic child" by Carl H. Delacato, he studied autistic children and his findings through observation suggested that Autism was Neuro-genic and not psychogenic as was predominately thought of at that time.

Sensory processing is a part of all of us, every nano second of our lives, every animal, plant, and human uses its senses to navigate themselves in and around any given environment. We are in essence sensory beings in every way you can think of.

Our internal bodies, also are sensory systems that tell us when we are hungry or full, alert or tired. They tell us when we need to go to the toilet as well as helping us feel our way around our bodies in relation to self and the environment we are in.

For many autistic people, sensory processing challenges, of heightened or lessened variants are an active part of their neurological makeup. Sensory processing Disorder (SPD) is a medical term and an official diagnosis that humans can havewithout being autistic. It is a stand-alone condition that can affect one or several senses throughout life permanently or temporary for a vast number of reasons. Equally you can be autistic and not have any sensory issues, although this is rare.

The term disorder is something I have grown to personally dislike. I prefer to use other terms such as challenges, differences, enhancements, heightened, lessened, or simply state which sense is super sensitive or under sensitive.

This book is written from the perspective of sensory processing when being autistic, from birth through child hood into adult life.

That said, Sensory processing is a natural human function. The difference is that the neurotypical human (generally) not absolutely, does so without any effort or discomfort, it simply happens. Only when incoming sensory information is extreme, such as a really pungent smell or extremely loud noise like a jet whizzing across the sky, does it become overwhelming, scary or even painful for the individual. Meaning only when that person's senses are pushed to their limit one way or the other— heightened or restricted that it is noticed or causes any challenge or concern.

I will be inviting you to take a look into your own sensory needs. How are your smell /sound senses? Are they heightened or dampened down in any area? Are there particular colours or patterns that create a negative response for you? Maybe certain pitches create an internal discord or a fantastic feeling of euphoria that either leads you to veering away from or wanting more.

I will be highlighting some simple, mindful activities for you to try. The aim is to help you focus on your personal sensory needs and functioning. You will learn new things about yourself that you perhaps have previously not given any thought too. Through observing your child's sensitivities, you will learn more about yourself.

They are your teachers, and they will help you to support them with a clearer understanding and compassion in how your child maybe experiencing and processing their environment in its entirety.

Something as simple as eating an orange can become a very different experience when instead of just eating it you take the time to smell each piece, taking one section at a time and let it sit in your mouth before you chew and swallow. By slowing down the process, it gives your smell and taste senses time to properly absorb the essence where you will have a very different experience, I urge you to try it.

Having some mindful quiet time, listening to the wind, birds singing or even the sound of traffic and isolating each sound one at a time can help you realise how dampened down your senses have become. You have a natural ability to shut out multiple sensory sounds and activities in any given experience.

How many of you have suddenly become aware of birdsong? When really the bird song was happening all the time, you simply were not consciously tuned into it. Often an auditory sound can be noticed once it has gone. Think about the ocean, have you ever gone to the beach, had a wonderful time, then left and noticed how quiet it is? It is then that you acknowledge how loud the surf ebbing and flowing onto the beach was.

These self-discovery insights will help you see how your child is experiencing the world, and awareness of your external and internal environment will heighten. Over time with this newfound awareness of yourself you will begin to feel a natural deeper connection with your child. Learning about your sensory map will begin to connect you with them through your understanding of your own sensory experiences and therefore feel an empathy with them.

In books about autism, and other articles or information you will come across the phrase "locked in their own world". This simple little statement causes a lot of concern for parents and carers which becomes the driving force to how the child is perceived.

Somehow, believing this notion creates activities and therapy sessions that dance around this idea. Creating a space where the child is looked at as needing to be pulled from some strange and mysterious world that nobody else can enter.

This is so far from the truth, Autistic children are in the same world as you, they are simply experiencing it differently. In fact, closer to the truth is an autistic sensory sensitive child is so engaged in the world/with the world that it creates the behaviours that are often seen as the problem. Once you begin to understand and reconnect with your own sensory experiences you will learn that your child is deeply engaging with this world, more than anyone you have ever met! Just because you personally cannot see, hear, or smell something, does not mean it doesn't exist. For others, experiences are very different, intensely so in many cases.

There are many ways in which a human can communicate with their environment. For autistic children, this can mean with their toys, although they will have an intended use and an "appropriate play expectation" as well as a suggested age range, your child may have a different way of using and enjoying that toy.

Play and how autistic children "do it" is for some forms of therapy— a concern. What I call "solution based" therapy such as behavioural led sessions particularly find play an area that needs to be addressed. A lot of focus is put into getting the child to "play appropriately".

This is a huge subject and one that merits a book of its own. For now, I will briefly explain.

Play is subjective to a child's neurological makeup. For some children, a "toy" becomes a sensational array of sound. The actual specified purpose of the toy is meaningless, instead the joy comes from pushing certain buttons that make a particular sound which may be extremely pleasing. Alternatively, a noisy toy may be excruciatingly painful and annoying to an autistic child who will instead disengage from it altogether, whilst the person who bought the toy sees only joy and excitement and does not understand why it causes either discomfort or holds no interest for the child.

This is just one example, as I have said play and sensory processing is a huge subject. Throughout the chapters I touch on play and how each sense may affect the play experience to give you examples of how the processing of each sense can manifest for an autistic individual.

Someone I came across a few years ago explained interaction with objects was a non-speaking, autistic person, her name was Amanda Baggs. She offered an incredible insight into her language. She was deemed; unresponsive to others, non-responsive to her environment, locked in her own world, lost and empty. How very wrong this assessment was.

She created a series of you tube videos, explaining and demonstrating what she was doing when running a tap and putting her hands in the water and humming. To the outside eye it looked like a meaningless activity, even slightly strange perhaps, in fact, she was communicating intensely and intelligently with the waters and the sounds, temperature and weight of it. For her, it definitely was not meaningless. It gave her great satisfaction; she was so connected to the water in a way that most humans couldn't even imagine.

Despite what others thought, she understood the cruel words that had been spoken to her throughout her younger life. She had been subjected to enormous amounts of abuse and cruelty in care homes. Despite this, she remained strong and more incredible, she needed to teach others "her language". Like all of us, she too had something to say.

I suggest you look her up, I promise you after watching you will feel very differently about any child or adult who is nonspeaking and likes to interact with their environments in similar ways to Amanda. She has since passed away, leaving a great wisdom behind. In a 20-minute video, she gave the equivalent to a master's thesis on nonspeaking communication, in my opinion.

She gives insights into physical movement and examples of herself doing simple tasks such as boiling a kettle. She shows how debilitating it is for her when a neurotypical person misunderstands her neurological and intellectual ability. What might look like mindless movements has, instead a logical and reasoning pattern to it.

Many autistic people who appear to be struggling are not given time to complete tasks, instead their carers consistently misunderstand them or have a predetermined mindset of what they are thinking, like Amanda, many were not even considered to think at all—in physicality, intellect or a communicative stance.

In her short videos, she shows exactly how wrong those people were, her intellect is obvious and her explanations of how her bodily functions and her neuro pathways are trying to match up to get her to do something as simple as boil a kettle are explained so clearly.

Watching her videos is not only an education but also empowering. It adds to the understanding of your child and how it may be for them in similar circumstances.

I will also be mentioning throughout the book how other areas of life, such as illness, tiredness and natural development can affect sensory processing for an autistic child, which can be either temporary, permanent, or fluctuating throughout their lives.

For the majority of neurotypical people, such intense sensory experiences happen in certain time frames. Take holidays for an example. Many a person has come back from a trip and spoken of the smell of the ocean and how the fresh air smells of the meadows and mountains. Food tastes better and they notice more about their environment. Is this because other sensory stimuli have been dampened down? You know, the hustle bustle of busy streets and busy minds, rushing here and there. Yet when on holiday all of that can be put on hold, leaving the mind to rest and simply focus on the experiences of the holiday.

Another factor is when poorly or over stressed which can create heightened sensory challenges or even dampen them down. The point I am making here is that it is when one is pushed to their limit, emotionally or intellectually that overloads happen and concentration is compromised.

In more recent years, SPD (Sensory processing disorder) has become a subject that is beginning to be discussed, studied and acknowledged as possible attributes to an autistic child's/adult being. From my understanding, experience and research, Occupational Therapists (OT) have the lead in this area of support.

My experience of this happened about 11 years ago when I was invited along to a parent/professional workshop on autism. It was organised and hosted by our County Council Educational Department. I went along with 2 hats, one as parent and the other as an early years professional and autism workshop provider.

The whole event, bar one session was, in my opinion, very disappointing. The delivery, information, activities, and language used was shocking to me. The workshop host gave basic explanations on the stereotyped findings of autistic children. The information and concepts were very outdated and lacked any knowledge that was either positive or helpful. I challenged the examples and the "advice" that was given to parents who nervously asked questions. I was, myself a parent of 5 years to my autistic son and had spent hours engaging with autistic folk of an array of ages and experiences. None of this matched up to my own experiences or what autistic people had shared with me.

The way in which the parents were being spoken to was saddening to me. Most were new to parenting and many had only neurotypical children, they were now experiencing autism for the first time. We were seeking and needing support, looking for advice that would give empowerment that could benefit our children. Instead, we were told that all our children were basically the same and to expect A or B to happen.

The irony of the first workshop was that the content did not match the experiences the parents were sharing with the group. One piece of advice given publicly without any substance or professional right was to medicate their child. I was shocked that someone who was not qualified to suggest that did so without any apprehension. More so they lacked any obvious awareness of the fear they had instilled onto these parents who had come to the workshops to become better parents and build a positive relationship with their child.

Before leaving that workshop very disappointed, I made it known that I was alarmed that such advice was dished out, like it was no big deal. I complained about the content of the entire workshop and how it was delivered. This was an event that was repeated across Wales and possibly other Counties in the UK. The audience was a mixture of parents and professionals across a broad spectrum. I felt it was important that this farce was stopped as quickly as possible. This could not continue to be accepted as training.

I moved onto the next workshop which was provided by the OT department, thankfully it was a completely different experience. I found myself being extremely emotional, in a mix of excitement and relief. Unlike the previous workshop, this one was speaking about sensory needs and overwhelm and how supporting this can help create a happier child., They were describing some of the possible reasons a child may be behaving in certain ways. How they may be experiencing the environment via their senses. Although this was a very limited amount of information, it was definitely a step in the right direction, because it spoke of individualisation, rather than a one-size-fits-all attitude.

This workshop was a taste of hope to me, I engaged constantly with the OTs during the 2 hours session. This got me excited and I was eagerly putting up my hand to add my personal experiences of what I had learnt from my son, others and myself. As I looked around the room, I could see parents smiling at what they were hearing, they could relate and felt their children did belong, that they were not the only ones feeling isolated and scared.

A scared parent is no help to a child.

Later that year I had a sensory assessment meeting arranged for my son—who at that time was 5 years old. This was a brand-new assessment, fresh off the shelf so to speak! It was a huge pack to be completed by me, his dad, and his teacher. Unlike the many other assessment forms, we had completed over the years this one was a joy! It was so much more detailed and asked questions that were more relevant to my son than ever before.

The reason the sensory aspect of autism and therefore behaviours (communications) are so important is that it enables the neurotypical person (parent or professional) to understand where the child is coming from. It helps to see the reasons why a child is behaving in the ways they do. This creates a bridge between you both, instead of a huge gap where many parents say they feel unable to connect. It also helps create a positive attitude towards your child's different way of being instead of others seeing them as problems to be solved.

You see, sensory reasons can create behaviours that can look confusing to the unenlightened eye. Looking at a child from the point of view that they need to be fixed, or what they are not doing in comparison to their neurotypical peers can create a lot of fear to the parent and therefore a feeling of disconnect. This can be catastrophic for the autistic child.

A common mistake is comparing an autistic child to the neurotypical one. This can lead to only one conclusion; your autistic child is wrong and must become more neurotypical to be accepted and to have any chance of thriving in life. I say, have more faith in your child and in yourselves.

I promise you that once you open the window of sensory seeking needs and the reasons why heightened and dampened senses create certain behaviours, you will feel much calmer and positive about your child's place in the world. Seeing things from the perspective of your child and how they perceive their experiences will make sense. There is always a reason for any behaviour, however odd or unfamiliar it may look or seem to someone else.

Being an adult and being misunderstood, with a voice can be tough. Imagine being a young person and feeling overwhelmed by almost everything you encounter. Add to that if you are nonspeaking, how on earth do you tell others how you are feeling or why you are doing what you are? You must show it through behaviours, there is no other way. But to have those behaviours interpreted incorrectly, often being seen as aggressive or meaningless, rude or "inappropriate" (one of my least favourite phrases!) can and has led to serious problems for the autistic person, such as depression, suicide feelings and attempts, low self-esteem, anxiety, and sadness.

I will speak about this in more detail in further chapters, also touching on how your child needs time to get to know themselves and how they filter the sensory input. Many of these methods are done physically or vocally, which are the very behaviours that can cause confusion or concern to the neurotypical person whether parent or professional.

Learning about the sensory reasons can show you a language never seen before and therefore those behaviours once seen as barriers or weird suddenly become meaningful. Every action and behaviour have a purpose, every sound is interacting with something or someone else.

Your child is different to the neurotypical child, whilst you can support your child to develop, being advised to expect them to behave non-autistic is unfair and impossible. Other differences in being human such as (for an example) Cerebral Palsy or Downs Syndrome does not mean they are expected to become non-Downs or non-Palsy. Instead, they are supported in areas they need. Such as communicating tools, sign language and AAC devices, physical aids and perhaps occupational and other supporting therapies.

A blind person is not expected to be trained to be non-blind…There is acceptance to their difference and any disability that may come with their condition, tools and environments are modified to assist that person's needs.

This is what the autistic child requires too. Your role as caregiver in whatever capacity that is, is to expect them to have their needs met with compassion and understanding. Insist that their needs are to be listened to and accommodated whether they are in school, nursery, college, university, family or work placements.

My intention for you is that once you have finished with this book, you will have the tools and confidence to do so. This isn't about becoming a Warrior parent or having to fight your way through a system. Far too many parents have had to do that (and still are) relentlessly fighting a system that isn't geared up to support their children because of a lack of knowledge and adequate training, as well as the right ratios of support staff.

When you have a sound understanding of your child's needs and can comprehensively explain this to teachers and family members, you will have no need to shout or fight to be heard. You along with many others will be doing the same. This is the time in our lives and society where changes are happening. There are 1 in 7 people (15%) of the UK population that are considered neurodivergent which includes your autistic child. This is increasing each year.

This means that you are no longer a minority in the family tree of "normal". There is no such thing as normal, it is a fallacy that doesn't exist, yet has created an illusion that has separated people throughout the world because of their differences. This is all we are talking about here. Differences.

Chapter 2
The Early Years and Diagnosis

As a Nursery Nurse (early years professional), I was a confident and competent advocate for the children and families I supported. I was passionate about my work, knowing in my core that it was my calling. My philosophy was all about child autonomy. I encouraged the children to lead and follow their interests from as young as babies. Part of my family support was encouraging parents to interact with their children in this way. The child's emotional needs and personal development was at the core of this practise.

I found seeing young children being controlled in their play activities difficult, even if it was good intended, (which it usually was). It felt far more beneficial to enable a child to take control of what they wanted to play and engage with. Discovering and exploring their environments naturally following their instincts with gentle guidance from the adults to ensure they were safe.

Throughout my working career I never questioned this, it felt right and it was having a positive and beneficial effect on the children and families I worked with. Predominantly, during those years (1988–2004), the children were mostly neurotypical along with some other physical and neuro differences of Downs Syndrome, Cerebral Palsy and what is known as Global Developmental Delay.

Looking back, autism was rarely mentioned, I can recall maybe 3 children in my care who would be regarded as autistic today. The work places I was in were in the mainstream and back then there were more "special schools" where autistic children were probably at. I remained confident and sure that my support and care was right for their individual needs.

Yet, as a new mother myself I somehow lost all that self-belief.

I think the expectations for myself as a parent was unreasonably high. After all, I was a trained early years professional—I should be able to know what to do to support my child.

Additionally present was the overwhelming input of other's opinions on how I should be parenting this little boy who was acting "very oddly" compared to "other" (neurotypical) kids.

There was a lack of understanding and compassion from others at parent—toddler groups and play activities in the neighbourhoods we lived in. Looking back, I know they were factors that built up into me feeling inadequate in the early days of my parenting experience.

I recall many a time going to toddler groups and sitting on my own with J when he was as young as 12 months old. I had to watch his every move, although not unusual for a child of that age he still stood out as different to the other youngsters in the room and the other parents noticed.

My confidence plummeted, my protection of J increased which became irrational and isolating. I really struggled with this as I am a social being, especially when it came to being around children. I enjoyed sharing with others in conversation and fun. After all, during my vibrant career I was always working as a team with other staff and obviously loads of children from differing backgrounds and cultures. We were a mini community sharing in the welfare and care of the families who came to our centres. This made for a happy and healthy atmosphere not only for the children but also the parents/carers and staff.

Suddenly I was completely alone. It was a harsh reality and one I simply did not understand, or contemplate. Emotionally this hit me hard, it felt so unnatural to be doing it alone! I was deeply hurt by the seeming lack of compassion towards J and me during those few early years of J's life and my new experience as a mum.

As a result, I believe it triggered old traumatic childhood memories within me when I was bullied daily in primary school as young as 5 years old. I wore glasses, had a patch on one eye, wore special shoes as I was pigeon toed and I was extremely shy. Mostly sucking my thumb and hardly speaking, wetting myself regularly and eating very little food.

I was quite different and at school this was highlighted especially to the other kids. Teachers didn't understand my shyness and constant need to use the loo, I was so nervous all the time. I often wet myself in class which was humiliating and worse still, the teachers back then would handle it by shaming me. That was their strategy to help me to stop wetting myself! This was around 1975/6/7.

I was either ignored by the other kids, laughed at, hit or teased, chased and generally terrorised, even some of the teachers were cruel as young as primary school. I never told my parents, I didn't understand any of it and so I clung on to my imaginary friend (until I was 10 years old) and spent my alone time talking to the moon, trees, flowers and animals. Yep, I was what was regarded as a weird child, particularly in school. I had two worlds, the one where humans resided, which I stood on the outskirts of bewildered and the other with all of nature and my imaginary friend, which is now what I believe to be my spirit guide.

By the time my son was born, we had relocated to rural Wales surrounded by nature, spending the early months of his life out in all weathers. We were extremely happy for a while; my life was harmonious and being a mum in our own bubble was bliss for me. Yet, despite this idyllic picture, the truth was that I was secretly incredibly anxious.

I had become increasingly protective of him, worrying constantly whether he would be OK. This was exhausting, scary and lonely all at the same time as I didn't express my feelings, instead masking them as I had done for most of my childhood. I tried really hard to not let anyone notice. When you live with someone in close proximity that is a difficult act to behold and J's father noticed, he would ask me what was going on and be as supportive as he could. He didn't understand what was happening because I never explained, I didn't know either. All I knew was that I felt a deep sense of fear that he would get hurt when not in my care or in my eye view.

Everything concertinaed bit by bit with all the isolation, worry, lack of sleep, disconnection, self-loathing and even more worry of not knowing how to help my son feel happier and safer. It had been slowly bubbling away and my sensitivities and struggles peaked from what was, for almost two years, an undiagnosed postnatal depression.

As my son grew in age, his differences became clearer to everyone we came across. Not just friends and family but strangers in the few social places J enjoyed which was adventure parks, swimming pools and activity soft play centres. This pulled us further and further away from the mainstream, including social events and meeting with friends and their children. It was very clear he was struggling with many aspects of the environments he was in.

At first, I had no idea why or what it was that was causing him to lash out physically which resulted in him banging his head onto walls and floors. He did this every day, throughout the day that resulted in him having a permanent bruise and cut on his forehead that I fretted about constantly. I had sleepless nights so scared he would not wake in the morning through the damage he may be doing to his brain, I wondered how could such a small boy cope with all this stress and anxiety.

He needed to put everything he could into his mouth. He sought it out, not like other babies who explore with their mouths at that age, no, he was seeking out stuff with an urgency and deep need unlike I had seen any baby do before. During my career I had looked after a lot of babies! Everything he touched went into or was passed across his mouth and tongue. He would lick puddles, water drips off gates, windows, toys, floors, anything he could. He was extremely happy one minute then boom, screaming and headbanging the next.

All of this intensified for him around aged 12 months and onwards, awareness of his surroundings was more prominent as it naturally is for any child as they grow and develop. This all caused so much trauma for him. The only things that gave him peace was being in nature, particularly water and also sleeping.

Living in a rural setting, support services were limited and a lack of adult company was a huge problem for me. We had already moved twice since his birth, each time hoping we would find some support and likeminded understanding.

When J was about 2.6 years old, I decided I wanted to move back to Essex to be closer to my family where I had a mum, 2 brothers and a sister as well as friends.

We moved back to a lovely little semi-rural village, nearer to family members and friends where we (I) felt we would get a better quality of life.

No one else in my family's history was autistic, surprisingly I at that time had never found a genetic link from any of my ancestors. I had never quite come under the category of autism myself, never myself considering I might be. I had been told by a couple of autistic guys I had dated that they felt I was. I did some online tests which always came out that I was borderline. It certainly wasn't acknowledged or considered when I was a child. (I later learnt that I had masked for so long I needed to unravel to get a clearer view of myself to complete such tests)

This meant no one in my family had a clue how to support this seemingly distressed toddler who acted differently to any child they had ever seen before. He could not give or accept cuddles or perform to the needs of the adults like other toddlers did. You know, the games we play with toddlers, singing, storytelling, catching and throwing a ball on demand. Many neurotypical children have no trouble being around lots of adults and noise.

My son was totally different, preferring to take himself off and be away from visiting people and relatives. My family were happy I had moved back for they had missed me and were keen to visit to spend time so they could get to know their grandson and nephew. However, J only coped with either me or his dad, anyone else he would ignore or run away from. This was confusing for them as I would invite them over for dinner or lunch and would then either disappear with J or his dad would, leaving them to entertain themselves.

Taking J to their homes or meet in restaurants was impossible, at first, we did but he screamed and cried his way through it. I remember packing up as much home stuff as I could to help J feel happier and safer in the different environments, but it didn't work. He would kick, scream and headbang at the door after about 20 minutes of being there so we would leave.

Although I knew in my heart J was autistic, autism was never mentioned at that time, not even by me. I was so tired and stressed out, using all the resources I had to focus on J and how to help ease his stress that to explain autism to others was too much for me to handle. I simply did not have the energy plus I didn't know much about it at that time so any questions they might have had, I wouldn't have been able to answer.

Although we had moved to a fairly rural part of Essex, it still wasn't Wales and the freedoms, we had there in terms of nature wasn't quite the same. On the plus side, there were more services available to us, like parent and toddler groups, albeit unfriendly ones. But the play barns and parks were much busier which created more distress for J.

Things were very tense and relations between me and my husband were struggling because of the stress of our new environment. I felt alone still, despite the best efforts of family members and friends. Although we knew J was autistic, we had no idea how to go about getting a diagnosis or even if we should.

We decided to find a nursery place for J to see if he could enjoy being with other children and lots of outside space. Maybe if he was in an environment designed for other 3 ½ year olds, he would feel happier?

To my amazement we found a lovely very small private nursery in a rural setting who were perfect. Super professional, caring, compassionate and supportive. Thankfully with my years of working experience I knew what a good childcare environment looked like and we found the jackpot straight away! I will always remember with deep gratitude the support they gave me and J. The management were lovely and his 2 keyworkers were the kindest and loveliest of professionals we could have hoped for. J took to this small nursery environment well! (Throughout J's life I began to realise for him it was more about the hearts and compassion of the staff, rather than the activities they provided. His sensitivities meant he felt other people's angst.) I will be talking about this and the empathy myth further along in the book.

It was during this time we started the diagnosis process. I explained how he liked being outside, adored all things to do with water, didn't use any spoken words and would probably put everything in his mouth. They took it all in their stride with no issues at all. As the month's past, they began to get to know both J and me better and we began sharing our thoughts about J's behaviours and why perhaps they were there.

Autism had finally become a discussion! I think it was because it felt like a safe space, of judgement, expectations or demands. I told them I felt he was autistic and wasn't sure (at that time) whether we should go for a diagnosis or even how to go about it. They said they would be happy to put in a referral to the psychologist for J to be assessed, this was back in 2008.

Before we knew it, I was given appointments both at home and nursery. A psychologist visited J in the nursey setting and observed him over a few days. She came to our home spending the best part of a day asking me hundreds of questions about his needs. It was extremely thorough and quite agonising to be honest!

The psychologist was lovely but the number of meetings that followed and the detail required with other professional agencies, was gruelling. Any of you who have already gone through this process will know what I mean. It feels so personal and exposing answering intimate questions about your child laid out for what feels like everyone to see and know! Privacy privileges gone.

After a few months, we were eventually referred where more forms were to be completed. We were asked to bring J to the hospital to meet with a consultant to be further assessed to continue the diagnosis process.

I knew this would be tricky, J had become increasingly afraid at being in strange settings. The stranger they felt to him the more challenging it was to be in them. By unnatural, I mean clinical, smelly, bright or too big he would resist getting out of the car let alone enter the building. I will be speaking about this again in more detail further along in the book.

We went along fully prepared with as many distractions for J as we could carry into the hospital. Honestly it looked like we were moving in for a week—we had so many of J's favourite objects (notice I do not say toys? Many of these items were random materials that J took a liking to, not "traditional" toys. I will be discussing this further throughout the coming chapters)

J coped reasonably well to begin; well, he at least entered the hospital without any resistance! However, within 10 minutes he was desperate to leave. Thankfully the consultant was a compassionate man, realising the deep distress J was experiencing he said he was happy for him to leave whilst continuing the appointment with me.

He knew of my professional career experiences and after a short question and answer session he offered me an assessment pack which consisted of 75 pages! (We now know that this is not unusual in the processes of assessments for various support entitlements) I had already completed a 70-page document for the educational psychologist a few months previously not to mention the Speech therapist assessment form, the Occupational therapist and the nursery referral forms. I felt my heart sink a little at the thought of having to complete another gruelling set of questions.

He explained that this pack was meant for the professional team to complete, himself included. This was the final part of the assessment before any official diagnosis was given.

He went on to say that due to apparent detailed knowledge of my sons needs he suggested it would be beneficial to complete the pack myself. He felt I would be able to give the information from an observer's perspective instead of an emotional one as a parent. (Not entirely true!) He made it clear that this was not normal practise, and I was to be discreet about the assessment pack. He said he felt that by me completing it a clearer and more accurate diagnosis could be made for J.

Personally, I feel that all parents/carers should be given such a pack and looking back I think the consultant did too. Hopefully after this book more parents and carers will feel confident and see they have enough knowledge of the child's sensory and emotional needs to do so. My tip is to add more than the question asks if you feel any tick box choices do not fit your child, write what does. Do not leave anything out.

I reluctantly took the huge pack home and began the long job of answering all the questions.

For those of you who have already been through the assessment process will know that completing these forms is a skill. I strongly recommend if you have not yet done so, find support to complete them. There is a certain criteria and language that is used and knowing what this is makes a huge difference in the diagnosis given and level of support suggested.

Help can come from Social Services and a variety of charity organisations—(SNAP) in the UK were brilliant back then and I believe still are to this day 2021, as are a charity organisation called Contact.

I was given a support contact which was suggested by the psychologist. You must answer the questions giving the worst-case scenarios, not lies or fabrications but the truth of how difficult things can get. As a parent this can be naturally difficult, a sort of natural protection kicks in and you find talking what feels like negatively is disloyal somehow. At least, that is how I felt initially.

When you have been living a certain way for a period of time, the stress and challenges become your normal, so you dampen down the impact it has on your child. I saw the positives in J, I didn't see him through the lens needed to complete the forms. I saw him through the eyes of pure love and so to tick boxes that highlighted struggles, disabilities and challenges was really hard. Even though I knew we needed support as a family to help him in life—expressing that to strangers and getting it right was very tricky.

I cannot express enough the benefits of you getting professional assistance in assessment form filling. PIP—Personal Independent Payments, EHCP—Education, Health and Care Plan, as well as disability living grants, carers allowance, blue badge anything to do with getting the right support for all any areas of their needs as well as the diagnosis assessments. J's social worker is always an excellent help and support for us with any type of forms we needed to complete.

Taking the emotion out of the form filling is hard but it can be done, especially with support this is where the agencies such as SNAP and Contact (UK only) can help you Actually, it is REALLY hard and looking back both his dad and me struggled, remember we were new parents as well as me having post-natal depression added to the now high expectations of the consultant. BUT once I realised, I had to slip into a professional mindset the process became easier. Do not misunderstand me, it was still challenging but definitely a bit easier.

(The difficulty behind completing arduous forms like this is because the language and labels used currently in the questions are outdated. In more recent times, Autistic communities have become deeply involved in taking back their power by becoming a part of decision making in policies for equality and acceptance. Although this isn't yet fluid across Britain and around the world, it is beginning to change for the better. Organisations such as governments, health and education institutions are playing catch up in what language is preferred by those whom they speak of. I will talk about this more in further chapters. For me, the autistic communities have become a huge part of my own empowerment not only with the raising of my son J but also for myself personally.)

The assessment diagnosis pack consisted of tick boxes and sections that needed short explanations along with ranking scores for each question from 0–10. The scores were added up at the end and depending on what number totalled would give you 3 different levels of an autistic diagnosis. Back then Asperger's was still a verified diagnosis that was seen as a different level to autism. This has long since changed and Asperger's is no longer deemed a viable diagnosis. This is an example of how Autistic communities and their campaigning has corrected terminologies previously used by the majority of neurotypical people and professional bodies.

Although this pack was more detailed than previous ones, it still did not give enough diversity in their choices. (In my opinion) Humans cannot be (or should not be) cooped up into small boxes of yes and no's.

It took us about 3 days to complete the pack which was now laden with our own notes and explanations and detailed descriptions of J in all the development areas listed. A couple of weeks later I was asked to meet with the consultant.

I will always remember this moment. I went along on my own, already knowing that J was autistic, there was no question. The official diagnosis was necessary to assist J in receiving the support he had a right to have when in school and throughout his life. Like I said the consultant was a compassionate man. He was very mature in age—I knew he had seen a lot in his career.

He smiled, thanked me for completing the forms with such articulate detail, he had never seen such accuracy in an assessment form, he said he found it incredibly helpful in feeling confident in diagnosing J correctly.

'I am very sorry,' he said suddenly looking very serious, 'but J is autistic.'

Silence followed as I processed his words. Silence not for the diagnosis but the apology he felt he needed to give me. As the bearer of such big news maybe he felt it was the right thing to say, the most compassionate perhaps. For me, personally, it felt strange. He wasn't telling me my son was going to die of a disease. I didn't need pity or apology for J being who he was, he wasn't sick! I replied, 'Please do not apologise for his diagnosis, this is a good day, now we can focus on J and begin to understand him and support his needs with clarity. Honour and focus.

I wasn't naive enough to know that some of our days would be challenging, gruelling even, we had seen how distressed J was already, yet I certainly was not prepared to begin feeling sorry for J being autistic, what good would that do him? How would that help us as parents to see his potentials, his magnificence?

He had challenges, huge ones actually and I was worried about some of his behaviours and obvious deep distress but being sorry was not an emotion I felt.

I was relieved we now had a diagnosis and could begin seeking support for him along with finding the most fitting of carers/teachers for his personality and individual needs. Suddenly I was empowered by this diagnosis, I felt my fire well up again, confidence started stirring in me, today was the beginning of new adventures, a different way of living.

As I drove home, I thought about the consultant's delivery to me of J's diagnosis. What if he had instead of saying, 'I am sorry, but your son is autistic' in fact started that sentence with: 'Congratulations, your son is autistic. He will be unique and super sensitive in many areas of life, enriching yours with new wisdom and strengths you never knew you had!' He will help you become freer in your own attitudes and thinking. You will live more in the now and learn about sensory systems in ways you never imagined. You will no longer sweat the small stuff, feeling liberated from the old paradigm of social rules and expectations that can keep you small in tiny tick boxes of acceptance.

You will learn that food is food, no division on what to eat and when it should be eaten, instead celebrating it at any time of the day! You will learn how to communicate using your bodies physicality as well as sounds and thought…You will experience profound moments of deep joy as you watch your child interact with nature and their environment that you cannot explain but just know it is beautiful and meaningful.

You too will begin to enjoy nature in this way, tapping into your own inner sensory system making you feel fulfilled, somehow more whole. You will hear his non-speaking voice through his incredible ability to express himself using his whole body, and as you become more practised in this you will begin to hear his symphony, you will feel proud of him and the human he is. He will inspire and empower you to become your true self, freeing you of constraints and insecurities you had growing up because you did not feel accepted. He will help you find your voice as you advocate for him and his individual needs and the needs of other autistic, non-speaking children.

Together you will walk side by side, knowing that every human being matters, actively contributing to society and humanness simply by being alive. You will watch your son be an active member of those like him who will boost evolution of human heart expansion and the celebration of differences in him, you, and all humans. You will see he is a part of those humans who are pushing through and eradicating the old paradigms of small-minded thinking and instead becoming expanded multi diverse thinkers in every sense of the word, yes Miss, congratulations are indeed in order!'

What if every consultant/doctor delivered diagnosis of a neurodivergent person in that way? Would that influence the parents/ carers attitude towards autism whatever challenges their children faced? Would it mean the dread and heaviness a diagnosis delivered with the words "I am sorry" would no longer exist? Would it empower parents to see their children completely differently from the get-go? Would it help you? I know that words are just sounds given meaning over time…Yet they do hold power, somehow on mass words are given power and then they become "truths" they hook into our psyches and become even more powerful, enough to completely influence how we see things and most shockingly, how we then choose to feel about our circumstances, worse still we start to feel less than, victimised and that impacts our children.

I left that meeting and headed straight to the supermarket, bought some champagne and headed home. As the cork popped the bubbles rose J's dad and I clinked our glasses and said, 'Well here's to autism and to J, let the adventure begin!'

Chapter 3
Finding the Right School and Support

Shortly after the diagnosis we decided that a move back to J's birthplace was the best thing for us to do. We preferred the richness of the rural land, endless rivers and waterfalls, empty beaches, rolling valleys and mountains.

J was and still is a nature lover, he adores being outside amongst trees and water. Water, in fact is his bliss place. He can naturally swim like a fish; under water for long periods of time, you can hear him giggling, his eyes open. I have no idea how he does it, he reminds me of the "Baha'i" – known as the water people in Borneo.

When J was young, his sensory needs couldn't tolerate a wet suit, he preferred to be naked in the wild waters jut as he did when at home in the bath or paddling pool. As he got a little older (8 years old) I managed to get a body warmer on him for his runs in the surf, even in January he wouldn't wear anything else!

Eventually as he grew and became more grounded (a deeper sense of his body and self within it) the coldness of the water became stronger and he accepted wearing a wet suit, I believe his love and need to be in the water helped him to bare wearing the wetsuit too. This was never forced onto him, I offered this until he was ready to wear it and thankfully, he did. He also wore water boots as there are a lot of jellyfish along the Welsh coasts, he needed to wear protection whilst in the winter waters.

Living rurally means there are fewer people but still enough to need to be aware of socially acceptable behaviours. We knew that as he grew and physically developed the general public would probably not appreciate seeing a naked child running freely amongst the waters and rivers. It seems to upset people! Imagine my relief when he finally did accept wet suits.

J has no natural awareness of his nudity and the offensiveness it can cause for some folk. In many ways, this is a wonderful way to be (in our culture) we tend to get upset over such things. Although I personally have no problem with his need to be naked as it is a genuine sensory led necessity for him to feel the most comfortable, especially when at home.

However, this can leave him open to vulnerability for being misunderstood, at a quick glance from a stranger they could become offended and see it as a public display of indecent exposure or even a flasher! He could be grossly misunderstood, possibly ridiculed or arrested.

J has an innocence to him still at 17, he doesn't care for anyone else's nudity either, for me as his parent it is both freeing and worrying at the same time. Of course, if we lived in Borneo with the Baha'i people of the sea it wouldn't be an issue. Culturally we are not set up to cope with or tolerate nudity.

I felt rural Wales would both feed and calm his sensory needs, he was happier with plenty of space and interaction with the natural environment. We wanted to live in a setting where he could freely and privately play in his garden naked. Plus, both his dad and myself preferred being in nature so it meant we could all get what we needed to create a harmonious family life.

We found a lovely home and headed back to Wales looking forward to new adventures and discoveries. I eventually found J the school that was perfect for him. This was not a straightforward task. My first port of call was a mainstream small village school with the aid of a support worker. Seemed easy enough! Haha! I was to find out that inclusion for all was not a reality. The words were bantered about in school policies and constitutions at that point (2009) However, this was not yet actioned. The right training was not made available (this is mostly still an issue across education and welfare for autistic children and adults in care) to teaching and support staff, yet new special educational needs policies were being implemented. However autistic children were continuously being misunderstood.

I phoned around the local schools within our catchment area, I wanted us to become a part of the community. At first, the Head teachers said they could cater for J; s needs and they had other autistic students in their school. GREAT! Then the reality hit home. As soon as I said that j was not yet toilet trained and needed 1-1 support things started to crumble. Adding in that he was not using spoken words to communicate made it very clear this was not going to be easy.

One head teacher said, and I quote, 'Well I expect that Mum and Dad will do everything they can to ensure J is completely toilet trained before he starts school here!' the truth was we had been supporting J in toileting practice on and off since he was 2 (he was now 4.5 years old). When I told him that this was all a part of J's needs currently and this is one of the reasons, he would need a 1-1 I was shut down. All children must be toilet trained before they start school!

Special needs policies, inclusive learning support and every child's right to education suddenly disappears if said child with a diagnosis and statement of educational special needs is not toilet trained. (I remind you this was 2009) This highlights that although new government policies were created that bannered statements such as "all inclusive" and created individual learning plans (IEP)based on the individual needs of the child as well as special needs policies, the training needed to fulfil such policies were not available or adequate.

Regardless of the lack of training and resources staff were expected to make it work. Therefore, the children, parents and teachers suffered, all feeling a sense of failure. This began to show huge cracks with parent/teacher relationships that over the years has increased to crisis point.

Another head teacher confidently declared they could accept J, until I mentioned he was nonspeaking as well as listing his sensory needs that require him to have a 1-1 support to assist him throughout the entire day. She commented on the noises she could hear J making in the background of our telephone chat. 'He sounds very loud.' I was surprised by her comment, as it's not unusual for a 4-year-old to be vocally noisy. I explained J, although nonspeaking did express himself through sounds. There was a pause, then she said although they would do their best, she could not guarantee that a support worker could be funded for J for full time education. (Even though he had a statement of needs which highlighted his need for a 1-1 throughout his school days)

Again, this indicated that School staff, including head teachers had very little knowledge on autism as well as the law when it came to Statement of Need (SON) Wales, UK and Education, health and care plans (EHCP) England. Additional Support Needs (ASN) Scotland, Child with a disability (CWD) Ireland. (As in 2021)

Please note that Education Settings around the world will have their own processes to assess a child's support needs and the abbreviations and labels given will be unique to that country and state, province, council, district etc.

We did consider home schooling for a while and if we couldn't find the right school setting for him that is what we would have done. I wanted to keep trying as he had been happy and thrived in his nursery experience back in Essex where he had a small number of children and plenty of staff, a huge outdoor space that all came wrapped up within a positive and compassionate attitude. He enjoyed being around other children, along with the experiences they offered him. Even if he didn't take part J loved and still does love to watch others enjoying themselves. (He does get pleasure from observing.)

I began to become disillusioned and felt a sense of injustice for my son's right to receive equal opportunities in Education. Right at that time our landlady told me of a Specialist School in the nearest large town to where we lived. It meant a 25-minute drive but it seemed like a good opportunity.

We went for a visit and I was impressed. It was a small school about 102 pupils aged from 4 to 19 years. The needs of the students varied some were autistic others had cerebral palsy, downs syndrome, ADHD, PDD, emotional needs and other health, physical and neurological differences. They had their own football team and took part in games with other schools in their community.

They had an end of year prom, discos, a business enterprise and much more. The classroom sizes were small and staff ratios high. They also put students into classrooms based on their individual and development levels instead of just age. Personality of the students was taken into consideration to ensure each student felt happy, safe and relaxed.

I was told by the headteacher that J could have a place at the school and start after the Easter holidays. BRILLIANT! That was super easy. THEN…

A week later I got a letter from the Local Authority Education Department telling me they did not have space at the school for J as they had what they called a Cap on school entries. How could this be? Why didn't the head teacher make me aware of this? I was confused, after all surely the Head of the School would know whether he could take J or not, so why was I suddenly told different?

I discussed this with the head who told me the politics regarding funding was a complicated one. He had created this school from scratch, cabin by cabin, bit by bit it was built and funded. His drive, vision and gumption were what got the school to where it was at that time. He had built up quite a reputation for himself with the authorities over the years he had created the school. He was a teacher who was to be heard! Which is no small feat.

If the school was genuinely full that would be understandable, except this was not the case. I was told by the head that there was space for J to attend and funding is available. He said he would support me in ensuring J was given his rightful place.

I decided to refuse the situation presented to me. At the time, J's dad was working in Essex all week coming home only at weekends to bring money in as we had not long relocated. Looking back this was a difficult time for me, it was energy draining to keep making phone calls, asking questions, fighting our corner and being told no over and over.

This went on for a few weeks. I decided to go to the local newspaper. They were interested in the story and a feature was created, a huge spread, photo and all. They came to the school where the Headtcacher, a few students and myself proudly posed for photos to support our story.

I was phoning every day for a month to ask to speak with the head of the education department and every day I was told he would either call me back or he wasn't available. I simply became a pain in the butt! I phoned 3–5 times a day, not just his department, others too—sending emails, copying in other members of the department and bombarding the phone lines. It was exhausting and emotionally draining. Eventually I got to speak with him, he informed me he was in meetings regarding this matter and would get back to me. This went on for another 2 weeks.

So, I decided to get the big boys in. I announced I would be employing a lawyer to assist with this situation. This was a breach against my son's right to an education. There was no reason why he could not attend the school from a legal perspective. I bravely stated to the head of the education department that if J was not given a place and a start date by the end of the day, I would be instructing my lawyer to stat proceedings to sue the department.

The truth was I had no such lawyer or the means to fund one at that time so with a deep breath and a huge prayer I waited. 5pm came, I started to lose hope…6pm came and still nothing. Where would I get the money from to fund a lawyer? 7pm…nothing. I began to feel defeated; I was seriously frazzled form the emotional energy I was using. Despite my wretchedness, I knew that the next day I would have to find a lawyer and the money to fund them.

Around 7.50pm that evening the phone rang, 'Mrs Berroyer, we are pleased to inform you that J has been successful in securing a place at the school and can start on the 6th April 2009.'

BOOM! I had no energy left to ask questions or to get mad I simply said, 'Good I will make plans with the school to settle J in first thing in the morning.' Just like that he was given the place which was already his!

The next day I received a call from the head of the school who informed me that not only did my hard work get J a place but it also opened up 9 other places for children who were told the same story as us. They too were starting school after Easter. This made me extremely happy; I had no idea that would be the outcome. To know that other families had benefitted from my pushing forward and continuous phone calls was amazing.

Now in 2021 J has attended that school for almost 11 years. We have seen 4 head teachers in that time and numerous staff changes. J has thrived during his time and he adores being there. They are like an extended family to him. He has been with the same teacher for 5 years which has proven to be of huge benefit to J. He has had a number of LSA (learning support assistants) changes but his main teacher has remained. As long as J thrives this will continue to be the case. Finding the right fit for our children is extremely important, it makes a huge difference to their happiness and ability to learn and thrive.

I remember J's first week in that school. Of course, I was anxious, he was extremely sensitive, non-speaking and semi toilet trained. His auditory senses were extremely acute making him sensitive to most sounds (and much more I later learnt, which I will discuss further along) and showed very little interest interacting with other children and staff. Although I felt this was the right fit for him, I did worry that I may be asking too much of him at that stage in his life.

I was hugely relieved when I met his first teacher, she was almost at retiring age, full of richness and wisdom. She told me in our first conversation that she asked herself the same question every time she met a new student which was, 'What will this child teach ME?' She practised this philosophy throughout her long career and boy had she learnt a lot. Through observing her students, rather than stepping in with a one size fits all mindset her students thrived at their pace and were all celebrated for it.

I felt instant relief—I knew she was the right teacher to settle J into school life. She supported me through a very anxious time, empowering me every step of the way. I will always be grateful to her for that. She knew that the children were her teachers, her classroom was always calm and joyful.

The advantage of a special needs school can be (not always) that the class sizes are smaller and staff ratios higher. This was certainly the case here. This meant the children had their needs met, they were honoured as individuals and time was spent forming trust between them. Every school is different, like anything else in life, looking around everything on offer will give you a clearer picture of what might be best for the child in your care and what their best fit is.

When I started out in my career, I employed the attitude of forming trust and positive relationships with the children and parents, especially the children. It takes time to get to know an individual. Our autistic children are no different, in fact it can take longer, because the complexities of a sensory sensitive child need time to be unfolded, to be revealed layer by layer.

This book is not me telling you how to be perfect parents or carers, I certainly am not suggesting I am or that I know it all. I am though, sharing what I have learnt throughout my life of both being a sensitive, neurodivergent person as well as working with 100s of children and being a mum to an autistic child.

J has been my ultimate teacher (not my ultimate stranger) as was the heading of that book I read many years ago. We are all strangers to each other, well, until we are not! The difference with an autistic, non-speaking child and a neurotypical child are plenty. The time scales needed to support them develop are very different to start with. Plus, their sensory needs and intricacies are layered and not always what is first thought to be. Time is needed to get to know, and understand them.

Equally as important is allowing the child to get to know themselves. This for me was like unlocking a secret that no one else seemed to know or demonstrate. If anyone did know and by anyone, I mean other professionals who worked with autistic children, I hadn't heard them voice this very important need, other than J's first teacher. Thankfully, J's teacher of today and the last 5 years also has this skill. It works every time and creates an unspoken trust that is vital when supporting an autistic student.

I have learnt there is no need to rush, to panic or bombard with endless hours of therapy. You see, all children develop with time. Yes, even the autistic children! (I say that with sarcasm). Many of you would have been told or at least, it would have been suggested somewhere along the diagnosis route that your child will not get as far as a neurotypical child. A list of what they would not be able to do is assumed from the get go, or at the very least developmental milestones may be possible but only if you engage them with an early intervention programme as soon as possible. A heavy burden of doom blanketed onto you before you and your child has had a chance to have a go at life.

For me, this is the tragedy, not the autism, rather that we are fed so much negativity, which I have learnt has been born from a lack of knowledge of what autism is and how it and the many facets of it can manifest in our children's brains and pathways of development. It is an unjust stance on all concerned and it seems to create more fear. This can then fuel a child/parent existence and fill them with anxiety and hopelessness.

Autistic children are entitled to a childhood just like any other. You as parents and carers are entitled to enjoy your autistic child's childhood, building memories of fun and joy instead of just therapy rooms, assessments and isolation.

I am not going to bang on about autism being a gift and our children's geniuses. I am not going to pretend that we do not have worries and stresses that can often drag you down so low it is difficult to smile. Of course not, being a parent can be tough across the board however our children's neurology processes life—it certainly is not a competition of who gets it the toughest.

Having a child who is nonspeaking, autistic and sensory sensitive is different to parenting a neurotypical child, of course it is. We all know this, wherever you are in your child's life as you read this book, you will already know that autism is still seen as an enigma by the neurotypical masses in general. BUT that does not mean we are all doomed and must become neurotypicalfied! (I made that word up.)

There is a place for you as parents/carers and a place for our children. Thank fully the autistic community is a gutsy one! Full of wonderful humans who think and feel in such a way that neuro diversity acceptance has no choice than to thrive and be seen. A community I am proud to be a part of and stand by my son's side.

We are in a time of deep change in our human existence and autism is a huge part of that. Throughout history we all know that anyone deemed "different" whether it be skin colour, sexual/gender identity or belief structure, disability or neurological differences have been ostracised, bullied and quietened.

No more is this acceptable, as we continue to evolve, we also expand our hearts and our wisdom. Our autistic communities through their neurological differences are as far as I am concerned at the forefront of this change. You cannot stamp out a difference just because it is not accepted or understood.

Although there is still much that needs to be done for autistic people to be accepted and thrive in this world, we are all tooled with much more knowledge than previous generations. The adult autistic communities and their parents struggled through with unimaginable isolation, loneliness and misunderstandings of their children's needs and differences as well as parent/carers need for positive support.

Now we have social media which has been a game changer for conversations, debate and connections. Facebook groups for one have a wealth of information and advice, support and real-life experiences that autistic people are kindly willing to share. While every autistic person is unique, hearing what other actually autistic adults felt and experienced as children into adulthood has definitely helped thousands of families understand and better support their children.

These communities are your children's communities, therefore they are ours too, whether we are neurotypical, autistic or neurodivergent in any way. Everyone needs help sometimes, parenting in many cultures is not done alone or expected to. Instead, it is shared and celebrated as an honour and sacred experience.

I can see this wonderful weave of support happening all over face book groups, there are sub section labelled groups for autism support, ensuring you will find a group that will fit your child's needs, offering the support and tools that could make a huge difference to your child's happiness by helping the carers, you, to help the child.

I feel that one of the biggest pressures comes from the need for our children to fit into "normal" which really means neurotypical society. Finding the right school and right teachers can be tricky, although not impossible. There are many aspects to an autistic person's experiences, some of the manifestations of behaviours of autistic people are found to be difficult to cope with for their carers and peers. Self-harming such as head banging, hitting self, walls or other people are all very challenging for the whole family. Faeces smearing, breaking house furniture and a lack of sleep will cause any human to feel at breaking point. My intention is to not ignore or belittle those challenges but instead help you gain the tools and a different perspective.

Looking into the sensory needs of your child in every detail can and will make an incredible difference to the happiness inside of themselves and make their living experiences easier.

Secondly accepting that a positive and happy human experience doesn't have to look like everyone else's. Autistic people are mostly happy in themselves, being autistic doesn't automatically equal being miserable per se. It is the environment that can cause the discomforts and distresses but mostly the despair and unhappiness stems from how others treat them being regularly misunderstood massively, not being given a voice of their own, second guessed, spoken for, or spoken over builds frustration, self-loathing and deep sadness.

My book is here to offer some ways of supporting autistic children, through the perspective of their sensory needs. I will show how, slowing everything down and avoiding comparing a child to another, (the latter can create a panic mindset and a competitiveness that leaves you feeling like a failure as a parent/carer.) mostly the autistic person will feel worthless.

The coming chapters are going to explore the whole human sensory system.

If you are reading this prior to your child attending a school setting, hopefully you will feel empowered and inspired to discuss with the teachers what your child needs.

This book intends to support you to be the parent/carer who knows and understands your child from their perspective. You will feel confident when attending any assessment or school meeting where you will be listened to because of your confidence and extensive knowledge in what helps them to thrive at their pace from the place they are at. You can help create the educational setting that autistic children need and deserve to have. More so you could be a part of the change for all children in an educational setting. We are all teachers and learners—passing on the knowledge of your child could benefit many others in the future.

Chapter 4
Compassionate Thinking and Awareness

Being a sensitive child meant I felt emotions very deeply, not just of myself but also of others. To me it was as normal as breathing and I assumed it was the same for everyone.

I did my best to disengage from what I found confusing, which was mostly my primary years in school and life in general. School though was the hardest place for me to cope with because I couldn't escape it. I didn't have the confidence and knowhow to complain about the bullying and unkindness, Instead I became like a little vessel of internalised trauma. It took a long time to emerge from me and realise just how bloody horrible my first experiences at school were.

I often felt like I was living in a dream, like I was in the wrong place or at any moment a curtain would go up and there would be an audience clapping as I and everyone else took a bow. Nothing felt real to me, maybe that was a coping mechanism I developed as a young child. I can remember feeling this way back as young as 4 years old but I expect I did way before then.

I do feel that being the child I was and how it felt was a major factor in my decision to be an early year's professional. I wanted to do my best to be the adult who could be a loving, nurturing and positive person in a child's life. I am proud to say I did become the carer I always yearned for myself, during my younger school days. I have always been an advocate for children, sticking up for them in any situation, always seeing it from the child's perspective. I still do, all I ever want is to see children smiling and laughing.

What helped me cope each day was finding nature and spending hours with the old horses who lived in the fields across the road. Talking to and grooming them with my hairbrush I would share my thoughts whilst washing them with old sponges and buckets of water. I wouldn't just play in the mud and pick flowers; I would talk to them too. I would hear the earth speaking and I could see it breathing. YEP! I was that weird…except to me it wasn't weird at all it was perfectly real and natural.

Nature was my friend, everything felt like it had a pulse, I now know of energy and life force, then I simply and innocently accepted it, I felt a part of it, an extension of it even. I recall not telling anyone else about my conversations with the moon, animals and environment, even the rain would have a conversation with me. I seemed to have a sense that no one else around conversed with nature like me, besides I had a "friend" I spoke to all the time.

My "imaginary friend" was the only part of that world my parents knew about. I am extremely grateful that my mum supported me in this, I think because I was so shy and had only one (human) friend, she felt that at least I was comforted by my "imaginary friend" so what harm could it do me? My dad wasn't so sure—he worried that there was something wrong with me but Mum assured him I was fine and I obviously needed her in my life. A dinner place would be set for her too. She became a part of the family.

I would spend a lot of my time in my bedroom with the curtains closed sitting on the windowsill staring at the moon, talking to her and asking questions. I would immerse myself in my dolls and teddies, seeing them as real. My intense imagination and relationships with teddies and dolls were definitely my coping mechanism over and above the usual play a young child has with such toys.

I did of course have some interaction with other children, at dance classes, the brownies and tea at their houses. Although the latter didn't happen much and when it did, it was more often than not an unpleasant experience for me. The dance classes and brownies only lasted a short while as I found it all so difficult. I was completely disconnected to what was going on around me. I did get to perform a dance on stage with a ballet group I was in. I must have been about 6. I had no idea what was going on! I ended up doing the whole dance wrong on my own whilst the other girls all danced together. The audience all thought it was very sweet but I was completely devastated inside.

I had one real friend as a youngster who lived a few doors away from us, she was a year older than me, our mums were good friends. We stayed at each other's houses, spending time together throughout the school holidays. I adored her, forming an incredibly close bond. She was always kind to me, we had a lot of fun together, creating games of shops and schools, putting on all kinds of shows for our mums, it was great fun. Thank goodness for her! Thinking about it now, she became like the Band-Aid I needed from all the school bullying and constant confusion of life. She was my anchor into the real world, the human world and because she was so kind and loving to me, I responded. As I write this, I can see that through her kindness to me I felt seen and so I came out of my shell (so to speak) I think she saw a personality in me that no one else saw. We wore the same clothes and had identical haircuts, even getting the same Christmas presents. Our friendship lasted this way until she went to high school a year before I did.

Although most of my early child school days were full of trauma and confusion, it is important to say I did have a loving mum and family. I was a sibling to two brothers, one older, one younger. Later at 15 years old a sister was born. For the early years of my life, there were the 3 of us. Our household was busy, my mum had loads of friends which meant we would often visit their houses where I would "play". Truth is, mostly I was just there, being led around by the kids. We went on annual holidays to Devon and Cornwall and spent time with our grandparents, aunties and uncles.

From the outside, apart from being incredibly shy and sucking my thumb pretty much all of the time, I seemed like a happy little girl. The truth was I was always struggling. I just found everything so exhausting and hard, emotionally. I would wet myself a lot during school and at home most nights I would awake to a wet bed, this went on until I was about 10, maybe older.

There is a reason I have told you about this part of my early life. I hid how I really felt from everyone. It wasn't anyone's fault—I just did. I do not know why, I was so sensitive and unsure about most things, I didn't have the confidence to speak up. I didn't really want too much fuss or attention. Yet on the other hand I desperately wanted to have more hugs, have more close relationships but I found everything so hard. I coped with 1-1 relationships and conversations but any more than that and I would get lost in the chaos of it all, sinking back into myself and simply going with the flow. Yet not really actively participating.

My point is I hid it well, I did what I now know to be called masking. I know my mum would have helped me had she known and understood the full extent of my struggles.

Masking wasn't something I knew anything about. I hadn't heard the term until a few years ago. I came across it in an autistic led face book group. I learnt that sadly, most autistic people had said they masked (especially girls) as children and many still did into adulthood in order to fit in or at least not stand out! Mostly to please others and to somehow have some peace. Although the latter became counterproductive. Pretending to be or feel something different to what you actually do is incredibly exhausting emotionally and mentally. It can and does lead to all kinds of relationship issues across the board. Including the relationship, you have with yourself. It can take years to unravel. I know too well.

Most of us have "masked" at some point in our lives (whatever neurological makeup we are) pretending to be or feel differently in order to please another. Most of us are taught to lie about how we really feel, not in an obvious way but slowly over time, we learn that being different can leave you vulnerable—open to being ridiculed, bullied, disliked and shamed. Somewhere along the way humanity accepts this as normal. Then as we get older, we become wiser and start to unravel that and begin to lose inhibitions and become more of who we naturally are. This can happen as late as in our 50s!

We then recognise the freedom in becoming the true us, it feels liberating and powerful.

What if we didn't have to experience any of that and instead always feel confident and happy to be seen as we truly are, right from the get go? Accepted without the need for changing to please others? As I write this, I can see that younger generations are beginning to step into their truth in numbers way bigger than when I was a child/teenager. This makes me very happy.

Imagine, being so obviously different (autistic) that every person in your life, including family wanted you to act and behave differently. What if every aspect of your life was met with a confused person not understanding you? Yet, insisting you change to fit into their regime: School, Home, Socially, Work, Friendships, Relationships? Even standing at the bus stop minding your own business, needing to self-regulate by swaying or stimming in some way but not being able to in case you were laughed at or worse hurt because it made "others" uncomfortable?

What if you were seen as a problem that needed to be fixed or cured? Imagine having adults speak about you in front of you in a demeaning way? Imagine hearing people discuss why you behave the way you do and getting it totally wrong, constantly misunderstanding you. Imagine being subjected to punishments and behavioural training (labelled as Therapy) because the adults around you are told by professionals that this behaviour needs to stop, regardless of the underlying cause, message and more importantly, the need for it.

For the last 200 year +, that is how autistic people have been treated. Most people who were born autistic or had neurological differences or disabilities of any kind would be locked away, those who were not were mistreated and misunderstood on a monumental scale. Horrifyingly those locked away were treated terribly—drugs, therapies, environment—all to somehow hide or change the way they existed.

Most of us at one point in our lives have experienced being misunderstood or wrongly judged and we all know it feels horrible. Well, that is an understatement, in fact all kinds of self-doubt and self-loathing develops before a child has reached adolescents. This can create an inability to connect with oneself in a positive way which enhances the challenges of building relationships with any other humans.

The impact this has in numerous emotional and mental aspects of a person's existence is vast. This then creates deeper isolation and anxieties that create further behaviours that keep others away from being able to support the autistic person. An on-going circle of despair.

So now try to imagine being a non-speaking autistic child and being misunderstood on a daily basis, right from the moment you are born.

As I look through autistic categorised face book groups, of which I am a member of many I see so many posts of parents speaking about how the school has misunderstood their autistic children. Parents who have to constantly meet with teachers who are told their child has caused mayhem in the classroom or they cannot accept this or that behaviour and are either punished or rejected from school. This is a huge problem happening all over the world, showing there is little knowledge or understanding of autism and how sensory systems are affected in autistic people, particularly children. Too many misunderstood children desperately unhappy who experience trauma and therefore develop post-traumatic stress disorder (PTSD) throughout their young lives all the way into adulthood.

During the writing of this book a TV programme was aired in the UK called "Please do not exclude me" it was about the current (2021) British education system and how children (as young as 6 years old, are behaving "disruptively" in class are being treated, some might say supported. Sadly, supported was not the case.

This highlighted the major lack of understanding of children's emotional and intellectual needs. More so the understanding of the child who is obviously struggling with the huge expectations for them to conform. It is clear to see the children featuring in the programme are neurodivergent—a system unable to nurture and support their needs. The loud message I heard was how the lack of training and resources which includes the ratios of staff to children is seriously inadequate.

Staff expected to perform miracles and get the desired "results" for the authorities and league tables (sigh) when the children's wellbeing and mental health is being supremely compromised on a huge scale.

Of course, this issue of misunderstanding an autistic child is not exclusive to school life. It filters into all areas of life including work places, family and peer groups and personal relationships.

All behaviours are communication and autistic children communicate and process their environment very differently to a neurotypical child. In further chapters, I will be explaining some of the many possibilities of why your child is showing certain behaviours physically, emotionally, intellectually and vocally. I couldn't possibly cover all scenarios as every child, autistic or not is different. BUT I can give an insight, a pathway into a number of reasons, when looking closely with sensory perspectives at the forefront of your mind.

There are many ways to see any situation, nothing is black and white—especially autistic behaviours. We are so much more complex than some of the "behavioural therapies" consider when it comes to autistic children and adults.

When looking at autistic children's behaviours, it is easy to have the viewpoint that life is deeply distressing for them and help (a change) must be given as quickly as possible. Like all children, some of this could be true. Yet not all of autistic behaviours are happening because of discomfort, some are simply a processing happening or a communication with their environment. Some are of joy and a need to feel their way around and, into the environment that they live. All of this will be explained in much more detail as you read onto further chapters.

On the other hand, there will be behaviours demonstrated because the autistic child is distressed, deeply. Screaming is seen as a very antisocial behaviour and is quickly treated as such. Yet for many young non-speaking autistic children, screaming IS a valid communication, asking/telling them to stop or disciplining them does not serve the child in any way at all.

What I have learnt is autism is not a condition that can be put into a box, completed and finished with a specific label. This is one of the aspects of diagnostic labelling that can and has caused both friction and mass misunderstandings. They can also create unrealistic expectations, depending on what "functioning" label the individual has been given at the diagnosis stage.

Autistic adults and more recently young autistic people have begun to challenge the many current "labels" they have been subjected to, from their perspective because of their own experiences of being autistic. I will be going into this further along in other chapters. The professionals who are responsible for issuing out the diagnosis are being urged to listen to the autistic communities to erase labels such as high functioning (HF) or Low functioning (LF), low, middle, high, grade 1,2 or 3, severe, mild or moderate autism. Instead, to be more specific in the individuals support needs in every area of their neurological, intellectual and sensory pathways.

Autism is a neurological difference that is far more intelligent than some of the existing labels suggest it to be, much more complex. It is unique in its design (if you will) for it challenges the neurotypical brain to think in a completely different way, often going against all child care books suggestions and behavioural therapy methods.

If behaviours are looked at from the starting attitude of it being "inappropriate" or "unacceptable" or "disruptive" or worse "attention seeking to get their own way", the child will always be misunderstood. It takes a loving and compassionate eye and heart to understand a person's actions and communication mechanisms. It takes time to sit back and observe a child's behaviours and learn what their sensory needs are. What is it your non-speaking autistic child is telling you about them and how they feel about the world and how it affects them internally and externally?

Observing with an inquiring and open mind, asking perhaps, I WONDER:

'What are they teaching me, showing me?'

'Why do they spin that way?'

'Why do they need to watch that same part of a movie 10, 20 times a day?'

'Why are they headbanging and screaming?'

'Why are they laughing hard at the water coming out of the tap?'

'Why do they not want to interact with me?'

'Why will they not look at me when I am speaking to them?'

The big question should be "I wonder how that feels to them?" And the even bigger question to ask yourself is, 'Why am I telling them to stop, before I know why they are doing…'

As parents, we are encouraged to ask such questions to professionals. While there are amazingly knowledgeable professionals out there, (many of whom, if you are lucky enough to meet, are actually autistic (AA) themselves) but if your professional team are neurotypical they will more than likely answer those questions from the only way they can, a neurotypical point of view and from any past studies and researches that were all carried out by other neurotypical people.

No one is more knowing about your child than your child themselves, the difficulty is when young they are unable to tell anyone the why's and the what's. Taking the time to observe and write down actions, patterns, cues, triggers and environments you begin to see answers, you really do.

You may not always be clear in your understanding of certain behaviours your child has, in time though you will begin to see patterns and behaviours emerge when certain experiences and scenarios take place. You will have a wealth of information ready to bring to the table when you have your first appointment with an outside professional such as a doctor, educational psychologist or psychiatrist.

Your child will need you to advocate for them with strength and clarity. They will need you to see them without the need or want to "fix" them. They will need you to accept that their way of being human is OK and to let go of the many social rules we are brought up with to believe is the norm.

It is important I think to remember you are not alone. There are thousands of others like you, parenting autistic children, all who are seen as different to the masses (neurotypical kids). Except when you really think about it, not so different for there are thousands upon thousands of autistic children across the UK and the world—vast numbers of whom you can connect with. With the help of the internet and social media, we are able to connect and support each other. We can share experiences and wisdom with "the masses".

Parents, carers and professionals can ask for help from autistic and other neurodiverse communities. I know there are an array of professionals who do ask autistic people questions to help them become better therapists and advocates for the children and adults they are serving.

The autistic adults I speak of are our children's community who were once children experiencing the behaviours your children are right now. It makes sense that you become a part of the autistic and neurodiverse communities to honour your kids and their needs.

There are conversations happening in these group posts that have previously in history never taken place. We are enriched with knowledge from autistic people who are willing to share their perspective and experiences. A direct line, if you will—into possible reasons and therefore solutions to support an autistic child's needs. Of course, EVERY child is different, autistic or not. BUT an autistic/neurodiverse brain and personal experience will give you an answer, a perspective that a neurotypical person cannot.

We need each other, both neurotypical and neurodivergent brains to unite. There need not be conflict and a them and us attitude. Both brain types speak and process language differently which of course can create misunderstanding.

Conversations between Neurotypical (NT) and Neurodiverse (ND) adults has it challenges too. I have seen conflict and defensiveness where both parties feel judged or manipulated. Equally I have seen some golden moments of solutions and breakthroughs with the wisdom and support of an autistic community member to a neurotypical parent and professional.

Speaking about our children and our parenting skills can leave us feeling wide open and vulnerable. Sometimes a typed conversation can be difficult to fathom. Was that sarcasm? Rude? Stroppy? The more conversations you have with autistic people, you will learn that unless it is stated clearly, there is not rudeness, sarcasm or anger—they are simply communicating in their own way. Direct and straight forward without the bells and whistles that a neurotypical person intends to need.

This is good practise to help you understand your own child's way of thinking. Autistic people speak in a more direct and clear way, they say what they mean, exactly what they mean…Whereas neurotypical people, often express lot of emotion embedded into conversations. Expectations of being empathised with from others to give comfort to you as if it is their responsibility to do so. This often creates friction between the differing neurotypes!

This is why I came up with the banner of "Learning the language of autism" I truly see it as learning a new language, just like I would Spanish or French. Like all languages there are many dialects—autism is no different. To the autistic person, a neurotypical person's way of communicating is alien and needs to be translated also!

Autistic adults on social media platforms are intelligent, eloquent and able to give arguments, conversing in complex topics, I have seen neurotypical people question whether they are actually autistic because they have read a stereotyped view on what and how autistic people (especially nonspeaking) communicate.

Many of the autistic adults who communicate through the social media platforms are doing so because they are typing rather than speaking or having to be face to face, using their AAC devices which creates a fast-typing mechanism to engage in faster paced conversations. When prior to such technology as internet, social media and AAC devices their voices were silent, no one knowing that, although different, their intellectual abilities were intact whereas for many previous years this was not considered a reality.

Many autistic people have enough "spoons" (mind space, emotional energy) to spend a limited amount of time on groups to chat and offer support. The rest of their day (as an example) could be filled with struggles regarding their own sensory needs or emotional struggles. Many have families of their own and jobs to attend. It is important for neurotypical people to be mindful of this. Just as it is helpful for autistic people to be mindful of the often (as an example) tiredness, overwhelm, worry or fear that a neurotypical parent maybe experiencing at that moment when typing a question or experience they need help with.

Now, more than ever in history (mostly because of social media) these differing neurotypes are listening to each other. This is creating the long-needed change to the wider world of human interactions and understandings of the autistic existence. We are a part of a huge mind shift and attitude towards our autistic children into adulthood.

Less talk of cures, fixing and changing autistic behaviours and physical needs and more talk of acceptance and real understanding.

Human beings are many things, but what we are mostly (I believe) is intelligent and loving creatures. WE ALL need to be seen and accepted. We may need to engage differently with each other, have different skills and pathways into existing and thriving as humans BUT we still all need and want acceptance.

The really good news is there is absolutely no reason why this is not possible. Of course, it is! All it takes is changing perspectives and letting go of the ego and the idea to be right all the time and needing to be on the side of a neurotype that is seen as better, normal or more than. When this kind of mindset is changed, the heart takes over and we see differences that can inspire us—help us be our own true self.

Children who are professionally supported need us to stand in the lane that is heart led, compassionate and unconditional in our attitude of acceptance. Let go of the fear of not fitting in, not reaching A or B development goals (for example) by a certain age so that they either fit into the school system or society that pleases others.

We are a continuously evolving species, surely the point of evolution is to become wiser, lighter, freer, learn from past mistakes, hardships, divide, be more heart led, and live more with unity and love?

The recent years of 2020 and 2021 has seen us all experience enormous challenges, every household and individual have experienced isolation with less human contact both physically and emotionally. This has stretched us to feel in our hearts with more compassion for ourselves and others. We are learning that community is everything and being accepted, seen and included matters to all of us so that we can thrive in our lives here on earth. We have put so much pressure on ourselves historically to be a "perfect" person. Are we, in fact, already each and every one of us individually perfect? Different, most definitely but perfect none the less.

This truth, surely then does not exclude the members of our human community who are autistic. Why is it that everyone else can be celebrated and accepted in their uniqueness but autistic people have to be "reprogrammed" into being or acting "neurotypical"?

Today's Neurotypical parents/carers and professionals have a wisdom and support available that no other generation have had before. With autistic and neurodiverse communities sharing their concepts, diagnosis testing and assessment experiences and ideas you can become knowledgeable about the children in your care. A true advocate with genuine understanding of their autistic and wonderful brains.

That has to be a good thing, right? The world is changing, humans are changing in every way. Our children have the right to be seen and heard, accepted and honoured just like all children do.

Let's dive into the sensory world of autism…

Chapter 5
Early Intervention
The Beginning of Learning
Their "Language"

As a parent/carer to an autistic, neurodivergent child who has sensory processing differences—you will be advised, most probably to get them into an "early intervention" programme as soon as possible. The logic behind this is to get an array of therapeutic programmes/sessions to assist your child in any developmental, behavioural and intellectual difficulties/challenges they may have.

Whilst this logic appears to be sensible, even necessary, there are some fundamental points that need to be looked at. The focus is to ensure your child is supported in line with their individual needs rather than that of others or their expectations. More often than not autistic children are expected to adapt to the environment rather than it being adapted for them.

Clarity of expectations is required to ensure that the child's individuality is supported in order for them to thrive. Highlighting their sensory needs and the necessity that they are honoured will ensure their emotional, intellectual and physical needs are acknowledged and supported also.

Additionally, this will help support your child learn how to manage and advocate for themselves in everyday life. From the get go, following this train of thought will keep all Individual Educational Plans (IEPs) and Education, Health and Care Plans (EHCPs) (or any Individual plan, report, target sheet, depending on your region and country this will differ in terminology) directly focused on specific and detailed needs from the child's perspective. You as the parent/Carer in their early years of life will be the only person/people who can help with this.

The term Early Intervention is used as a positive problem solver of all your autistic child's problematic (from others perspectives) characteristics. This often focuses on the behaviours first and sometimes (although not nearly enough) secondly, their emotional and sensory needs. Currently Occupational Therapy (OT) seems to be the lead and closest to recognising and supporting children's sensory needs.

A young child who is autistic, let's say as young as two years old will be very different to their 4, 6, 8 and older selves. What I mean by this is that a newly diagnosed two-year-old autistic child who has a variety of sensory processing challenges will develop like any child does. The process, though, will be very different to that of a neurotypical child, ensuring you acknowledge and accept this fact is key. It is easier then to accept that using the same strategies implemented to neurotypical children will not have the same outcomes for the autistic and other neurodivergent children.

Often things can change in time as your young child develops and becomes more experienced in themselves. Having their needs met can help them become stronger and more able to cope with issues they could not when younger. Everything is a stepping stone to something else. I have learnt this as a very valuable factor in my son's life and development. It is so worth taking the time and doing things the way they need it done, however that looks to anybody else.

What is one person's joy is not another's, this is an important point to remember about your child. They may not engage with experiences in the expected way or how the neurotypical children do. Instead, they are enjoying and engaging in the experiences their way—a way in which they can process the information being shared as optimally as is possible for them at that time.

There are many examples of this, some are; avoiding giving eye contact or looking in the direction of the speaking person (teacher) for example. Maybe your child needs to move around or stay standing up in a classroom setting when everyone else is sitting still? Maybe they need to stim in a way that can look like they are not listening? Perhaps they need to stand whilst eating any meal and use their fingers rather than utensils. These are vital traits which will benefit the needs of your child when you accept them as so. Passing this factual knowledge on about your child to teachers and other professionals who may interact with them into adult hood is the important role you play.

You can help change the old paradigm of autism behavioural understanding into the modern neurodiverse acceptance of what autism and sensory processing really means for the autistic individual you are supporting.

These experiences and processing needs can alter and fluctuate as your child grows and develops. Now my son is 17 he takes part in more activities than when he was 10, 6 and 4 years old. BUT he still has many experiences he prefers to stand back from and now I know why. I make sure others understand this so that he can be given the space to watch. If he does want to interact, he will. He has gained plenty of self-learning throughout his life within his sensory systems to feel confident enough to make those decisions for himself.

My role is to ensure that the carers around him know this of him too. I act like an interpreter of his language. Just as if he was speaking French to an English-speaking group of people—they would need an interpreter. As he is a non-speaking communicator and instead a physical, sound and movement communicator, an interpreter is necessary until they are fluent in his language.

As I have previously mentioned, a phrase that is regularly written and stated is that the autistic child/adult is lost in their own world, unreachable and lonely, so pulling them away from that and into close interaction with others is necessary for them to feel better. This is completely inaccurate and untrue.

The autistic person you care for is in absolutely the same world as you. All they are doing is experiencing it through different pathways. In fact, closer to the truth is that their experience of the world is far more intimate than a neurotypical person could possibly imagine. The interaction so deep and intricate that nothing is missed. This is often (not always) the reason why many autistic children do not engage with people, including their parents/carers. They are far too busy with the chatter, sounds and vibrations of their environment as well as their own internal sensory systems.

I will use this comparison as an example: throughout the world humans speak different languages, all with an array of dialects. At first, hearing a language spoken different to your own is baffling and it remains so until you learn some of that language. How do we do that? We listen, we watch and we learn, the easiest way to learn is to immerse ourselves in the culture. Of course, we can go on courses and read books, listen to audio tapes and so on. Putting yourself right in the culture and spending time with those whom language you wish to learn is somehow a more wholesome experience. Learning to speak and understand the language and all its nuances is easier, you get to understand contexts and complexities you may not have learnt from reading a book. Suddenly the language becomes richer and less forgettable because you can internalise it, rather than it being an external learning.

Autism is no different—watching, listening and immersing yourself without judgement and expectation of what your neurotypical brain wishes it to be, will enable you to learn much more about the child or adult you are supporting.

The younger the child often the more heightened their sensory experiences, both internally and externally. This is also because they have not yet found ways to filter certain sensory experiences which feel more comfortable to them. Therefore, their behaviours are more likely to be deemed as (my least favourite label) "inappropriate" and flagged as needing to be eradicated as soon as possible without considering their emotional needs and rights.

Whilst in some cases such as self-harming or unhygienic behaviours such as faeces smearing/eating/throwing, eradication can logically be seen like a good idea. However, both the methods used and reasoning behind them need careful consideration. This is not suggesting that they are left to continue smearing faeces all over themselves (for example). However, finding out why and investigating this deeply (there is always a valid and logical reason) will help you (and them) find a healthier and safer alternative.

Sensory needs are intense and usually a part of the autistic's experience, the two often go hand in hand, you cannot separate them no matter what methods are used. The dangers of either ignoring or being unaccepting of sensory needs are incredibly damaging to the autistic person. These needs can be pushed further away into their bodies creating anxieties and depressions filled with despair and loneliness. This can seriously interfere with the relationship and knowledge they have with their own bodies, often leaving them almost afraid of themselves, including the environments around them.

What can happen during Early Intervention Programmes that are behavioural based (EIPs) is the removing of the unwanted (by others') behaviours through bribes, prompts, punishment, repetitious language, stopping physical actions such as stimming and using time outs as a coaxing strategy. This is to be avoided for the reasons I have mentioned as well as more I will highlight further into the book.

My earlier point about age is that most autistic children aged under 5 years old (often older than that) are busy experiencing the world around them on an extreme scale without any filters. Although not all—it's very common for autistic children to have multiple sensory heightened or dampened down pathways which will continue into adulthood.

Being so young will usually mean they have no way of understanding what's happening with their bodies and internal systems or why. Therefore, they will not yet have ways of filtering out or have techniques to help reduce any unpleasant or painful sensations and experiences that are happening through their senses.

All of this takes time through repetitious experiences, amongst many other interactions which is best led by the child/adult themselves. Allow them the space to make their own choices in their own time and space.

Whilst currently there are methods used around the world in therapies that claim to cure what is deemed as severe unwanted behaviours quickly (such as ABA), the danger is they often ignore the child's emotional needs and just as important, their sensory processing pathways—which are a major reason why such behaviours exist. ALL behaviour is a communication of, or with something. This includes environment, an element, objects, people; basically anything, all sensory experiences are felt throughout the whole body which includes emotionally too. This is a very important point to remember if you are not already aware of this as it explains the intensity in the experiences.

The early intervention I am speaking of is to look more deeply, through a different lens other than the behavioural problem one. Usually when using a behaviourist's tunnel vision approach the only person/people who benefit are the implementers as well as everyone else around the child. Sadly, not the child themselves.

The purpose of therapy in the true sense of the word is to help a person feel happier within themselves for themselves—rather than looking and acting satisfactorily better than before therapy to full fill the judgement of others' expectations and needs.

Another important point to remember, although it seems obvious is that your child will become an adult. This means they will become bigger, stronger, more complex and if supressed in their early years, can become severely depressed—a shadow of whom they could have been. They may "behave well" in accordance to everyone else's needs and expectations, yet their self-worth and ability to self soothe and manage their own sensory needs will become non-existent.

No amount of "behavioural therapy" based on reward systems and endless hours of intense interaction can support their mental health and emotional wellbeing. The freedom to be able to express themselves without being judged and controlled can disappear over the early years of their childhood. Giving your child the space to learn about who they are and how their bodies react and respond through their sensory needs and their environment can be lost forever.

Some Early Intervention Therapy Programmes such as Applied Behavioural Analysis (ABA) sometimes known as Positive Behavioural Support (PBS), can include anything from 10 up to 40 hours + a week. A combination of school/nursery/preschool/Kindergarten and home settings. Every space your child is in is consumed with a therapy session of some kind. This leaves very little or no time for processing and simply being, living and having a childhood to explore and play in. Rather than a therapy to help support a person it becomes more in line with conversion therapy instead.

There is a lot of research on the internet with more detailed information on both ABA and PBS and why Autistic Communities are adversely against this kind of intervention. Many have experienced this kind of treatment as children and are now telling their stories to help prevent other children from being subjected it. Their aim is to have this particular therapy banned from the UK and around the world completely.

I speak of this because this was and is still currently suggested as one of the top Early Intervention Programmes to embark on. Before you do, please strongly consider the philosophy and intentions behind it and listen to what the autistic communities are saying about them.

Please understand I am not suggesting you go into an anti-therapy stance, far from it. It may become an integral part of your child/adult/client's life for a while. I am highlighting that hour upon hours, year after year (most likely) can become very distressing and harmful for the person enduring it. Taking the time to research and ask plenty of questions to both the people who have experience of them and the therapy people themselves.

Just because a person is autistic does not deem them automatically valid for therapy.

There are vast numbers of autistic people who have had no "therapy" and have developed and thrived in their lives at their own pace with positive and compassionate support from a variety of people and organisations. There are others who have the type of therapy that honours their needs and aids their life in a positive way. Others have had "therapy" for the 10–40+ hours each week for years of their child hood, into adult life a continuum of intense invasion of their space and thought processes.

A crucial and most important aspect of an EIP (Early Intervention Programme) is of you (the carer/parent/professional) observing and listening to the child's behaviours from a sensory perspective. Acknowledging this is crucial to building a harmonious relationship between the neurotypical (you) and neurodivergent brain functions.

This isn't about changing or reprogramming their behaviours or to act differently in accordance to social expectation. Instead, it is requiring you to observe them with the question forthright in your mind, 'What is this child communicating and why?' This way you will learn why they behave the way they do. By taking this action of observation, you are accommodating their need to express themselves whilst they process their experiences in a way that will help them to reduce as many anxieties and physical/self-harming behaviours as they need in order for them to feel happy and to thrive.

Another point to consider is that many (not all but a surprisingly large amount) of physical and vocal actions and sounds (stimming) are in fact joyful expressions—a way of filtering the vibrations they experience. Rather than the common assumption that they are negative, harmful or sad outbursts.

This is to all be figured out by you (a form of translation of their language). As their carer/parent or professional support this is an important role and responsibility that you have. An opportunity to positively support this person not only when they are children, but for the rest of their lives.

This type of early intervention looks differently to the mainstream idea of it. This version is more observation and recording down what you learn, the mainstream is about actioning changes almost immediately.

The early intervention I am speaking of, in many ways is the total opposite to the mainstream concept. Instead of getting into their (autistic child/adults') space and providing them with activities and intense interaction with you or using activities that force eye contact (for one example) or compliance to behave in one way to receive a reward we use observation and support through the sensory lens viewpoint.

This alternative method of observation and accommodating the sensory needs will assist in eliminating any experiences and feelings whether they are environmental or physical which can result in feeling overloaded and over stimulated into meltdown, self-harm, running away, screaming, crying and many other physical behaviours that are deemed unacceptable, or are harmful, painful to the individual. All of which are in fact intense interactions and responses to their environment.

I know I am repeating the need to observe; however I do feel it necessary because it can be such a difficult thing to do when surrounded by others telling you to do something else.

This may seem like terrible advice. You may feel yourself that to not stop such intense responses will only make your child continue to act in this way. Behavioural therapists may tell you that to do "nothing" will increase these behaviours and enforce their inability to connect with you. This is simply untrue. The one tool you need in these early intervention stages is observation through a sensory perspective. Trust me it reaps benefits long term for your child for a variety of reasons, some of which I have listed below.

- This method can create trust between you both in a deep and meaningful way which will enable you to introduce new experiences to your child as they grow and develop at their pace, them knowing you have their needs met and honoured.
- You will learn their individual language of interaction with their

environment and why they do so.

- You will learn why they behave the way they do to everything they experience. It is harder to do that when you are physically too close to them.
- You will learn how to slow down and appreciate your child's uniqueness and interactions.
- You will learn more about yourself and your own sensory needs by watching your child engage with the world from a sensory perspective.
- You will feel empowered and confident when speaking with other family members and professional departments about your child's needs and personality.
- You will be clear in informing family members how you expect them to interact and communicate with your child in accordance to their needs.
- You will bring valid clear advice and support strategies to assessments and IEP EHCP meetings for your child to thrive in any education/care setting you choose.
- You will have a wealth of sound knowledge and understanding of your child's behaviours, what triggers them and how you can help them to self-regulate.
- Your child will be free to learn about themselves before anyone overtakes and forces them to ignore their own sensory systems and fit into what others want them to do.
- Your child will learn strategies naturally that will help them cope with any sensory overloads or difficulties.
- Your child will become less afraid of new activities and experiences as they grow and develop because they have not been constantly overwhelmed in every aspect of their young lives.
- They will be more able to learn at school (for example) if their sensory needs are understood and accommodated to reduce stress and anxiety—ensuring they have equal opportunities to learn academically if they choose to do so.

- You will form a relationship and communication with your child that you never before thought was possible.
- You will learn new skills in how to communicate using non-speaking methods.
- You will learn that there are many aspects of being human (neurodiversity) that are valid as well as the neurotypical way.
- You will feel less afraid for their future because you will begin to educate others about your child, those people will then educate others and so on, therefore supporting the many other sensory sensitive autistic children in the world.
- Your child will have their needs met and therefore they will feel valued and as important as their neurotypical peers.
- Your child will learn that being different is OK.
- You will help your child learn about themselves and therefore learn strategies and coping mechanisms for many areas of their human existence, life long, not just for school.
- You will help your child feel comfortable to stim and self-regulate and ask for such space if they need it moving forward in their lives.
- You will increase your child's self-esteem and self-identity by accepting their differences.
- Your child's health and emotional wellbeing will improve because of decreased stress levels.
- You will accept yourself and your individuality more easily increasing your own self-esteem.
- You will confidently translate your child's language of non-speaking (if they are so) to others who share your child/adult's life.
- You will learn about non-speaking methods of communication such as AAC's (Augmentative and Alternative Communication) devices, as well as physical and sound communication.

This is all about learning their sensory needs by observing carefully through the lens of wonder and curiosity instead of just seeing a behaviour that has to be stopped. As you learn more about the child or adult that you support you can start to change the environment to reduce stress and overwhelm.

The symptoms (behaviours) that cause the pain or anxiety stress/overwhelm will begin to reduce as their environment is created to align with their individual sensory needs. As you read each chapter you will begin to understand how this Observational Early Intervention (OEI) concept works.

This will be an ongoing process as your child develops and grows as well as when their needs change. While some of their sensory needs and strategies may always remain the same, many will become less prominent. New sensory challenges may arrive through age, particularly when reaching the puberty stages for all genders. Through the development stages of growth and age often one's awareness of the environment becomes intensified.

For example, babies from birth—3 months will be less aware or affected by the outer stimulation of their environment (although not completely) some of their autisticness will be missed by the adults purely because a baby's behaviours are expected and accepted as normal development. Babies will stare "into space" and will move their tiny arms and hands in repetitious ways and make random sounds. They may sleep or blink a lot for example, this wouldn't at such a young age be considered different.

My main point here is there is no need to rush things along. This is what the ABA and PBS therapies tend to focus on with the hours upon hour of repetition to get the desired outcomes and behaviours as soon as possible. This may be seen as necessary in order for the child to "fit" into school settings or what social expectations have, however it may not be helpful to the child/adult you are supporting.

The child you support will be your greatest teacher, if you are open to learning—your role is to observe then accommodate their teachings.

All behaviour is communication, self-harming and vocal sounds of any kind are ways your child/adult is communicating their experiences and needs. Some are simply expressions and interactions of what they are engaging with. Some sounds and actions are conversations they may be having with everything they see, hear, smell, taste, touch or feel. Anything and everything such as water or colours, textures, nature—objects of any kind, including their own bodily functions, feelings and emotions.

Their physical behaviours that are self-harming may also be a conversation with whatever it is that is causing them to hit or bang or scratch themselves. It could be painful or joyful, it could be their way of filtering out or down or waking up the intensity of any such sensory pathway at that time.

Another important point is these reactions and responses, however extreme they may look or seem to a neurotypical person are not a choice. Rather they are a physical reaction to the input they are receiving initially but more than that it is a complete emotional and physical experience to the core of their being. The intensity of these sensory experiences can interrupt the ability to think, speak, see, smell, taste and function in what society sees as "normal" or easy.

It is important to say that you will probably misinterpret many behaviours, make mistakes and feel out of your depth sometimes. Learning such things does take time. Try not to be hard on yourself or give up, being honest to your child will help you both. If you feel or can see you have made a mistake, tell your child, apologise to them and start again. This is definitely not a mistake free process. Learning about another person's sensory needs and language when they are so complex and intense isn't a 5-minute job.

Autism is a high intelligence (that's how I see it) it is so intricately detailed. An autistic, will feel everything deeply, internally and externally without a choice or a decision process. Autism is a neurologically different way of experiencing life to how a neurotypical person does. There is no cure and it starts at (pre-birth) birth and ends at death.

Accepting this fact particularly for parents of young autistic children is integral to a happy family life and fulfilling relationship between parent/carer and child. If it isn't accepted as such or years go by where the parent/carer is hoping for a breakthrough cure of some kind to make the child non-autistic, the more painful and exhausting this is for the autistic person. Them always knowing their parent/carer wants them to be different and them knowing they never can be.

Nick Walker is an autistic PhD guy who has given an explanation on what autism is based on science rather than a social concept. It is a very clear, up-to-date explanation that diminishes any old, untruth myths about autism. He is easy to find if you search his name online, he has YouTube videos too.

I do understand first hand any parent/carer wanting the best for their children. Of course, I do too. Their happiness is paramount, this is exactly what this observational approach is all about. Finding out what does make the autistic child happy—it probably will not match what you think creates happiness for them.

Helping to advocate for your child by learning about them truthfully from their perspective will absolutely create happiness for them, not only when they are children but way into adulthood. Being nonspeaking or moving and flowing through life using sounds and movements doesn't mean they will be miserable. Being misunderstood or spoken for, ignored and disregarded are what creates unhappiness and loneliness for that child.

It is documented in some books and papers that somehow being autistic is a separate part of the child/adult, as in the phrase "has autism" as if it doesn't define them. Yet in truth it does. Being autistic is a wholeness like any other neurological state of being is. Humans have many definitions of self, don't we? I identify as a woman, I am a writer, a mother, a daughter, a friend, an empath, a healer, a dancer, neurodivergent and all of these things define me. Being autistic is in all aspects of thinking and feeling it isn't a separate part of a person like, say a temporary graze or a spot/pimple is or a cold or disease. A person can be autistic and a father, husband, partner, teacher, brother, son, nurse or acrobat—whatever! Defined by many aspects of how they choose to live, being autistic is all included within those aspects just as being neurotypical is.

Denying that autism defines someone can create a negative overtone towards the neurological system that person has as well as their self-esteem and mental health. Being autistic, means you are incredibly sensitive and the awareness of others disappointment is inescapable and can be soul destroying.

Many autistic and neurodivergent adults I have spoken and engaged with over the last 17 years have said when they were children their behaviours and sensory experiences were way more intense than when becoming adults. Please do not misunderstand me, I am not saying that once an adult any challenges and sensory overloads disappear. Definitely not! The difference is that most autistic adults (not all) have learnt how to self-regulate and decompress. They have had a lifetime of learning about what they do and do not need to feel comfortable in life. They have learnt what their triggers are and why. Autistic children develop just like any other child does, they simply do it differently.

The early intervention I speak of will help the carer/parent to learn the language of their child on many levels. I am not ignoring that there are times when things can be difficult. If an autistic child is having a hard time coping with something or sleep is affected or eating and bathing are all terrifying or difficult for them to name a few scenarios, it can be challenging. Sleep deprivation is no joke and it makes everything harder to cope with. The many aspects of a stressed out or overstimulated, sensitive autistic child can be difficult on a daily basis. I am not ignoring the realities of tiredness, peer pressures, family pressures, working and finding childcare etc. In fact, it is because of the many difficulties I read about from families with autistic children as well as our own difficulties, that I write this book.

The sensory needs of an autistic child are the gateway to learning so much about their personalities. It has to start there; I have seen them ignored time and time again. Instead, the focus has been on behavioural strategies alone and it usually ends up in despair for all concerned but especially for the autistic person. So many young autistic people become a shadow person of themselves, broken down because of being consistently misunderstood.

Mostly the key to a successful and beneficial Early Intervention Process (EIP) is:

- Letting go of comparing your autistic child/adult to neurotypical children/adults.
- Accepting they have a different neurological system in every way.
- Let go of fear and panic (easier said than done but it is possible)
- Watch with all of you (eyes, ears, heart)
- Focus on finding what creates their behaviours through the eyes of a sensory lens.
- Accept that their behaviours and responses to the environment are real and valid.
- There is not a need for attention (attention seeking) from your child/adult when they find certain situations overwhelming—in fact as their awareness of others grows with age—the attention of

others can be painful.
- There behaviours are not personal to you.
- Meltdowns/crisis moments/overwhelm are not temper tantrums—they are incredibly exhausting for the autistic person to endure and intensely upsetting.
- Their sensory overwhelm and behaviours are not a choice.
- Helping them to find a variety of ways to communicate their needs and wishes/opinions and thoughts as they grow and develop—more so accepting when they reject a particular method and help them find one they are happy with.

After observing, listening and learning through this method it may be that therapy is required to assist the person. Hopefully you will have clarity of what type would best suit your child/client. You will begin to be able to use a personal approach that aligns with their individuality, personality and needs. Finding the right fit in a therapy method, the therapist's personality, the hours offered and the environment.

My son has had some Occupational Therapy (OT) when he was very young and speech and communication therapy on and off since he was 4 years old. This has mostly consisted of me being given tools and resources to use with him at our leisure. This is just one example of what an autistic, sensory sensitive persons "therapy list" can look like. Do not assume autistic, naturally equals hours of therapy. By overloading the therapy, it is difficult to know whether that child would have developed certain skills overtime without it. Such as spoken language or interaction with peers or parents and developing self-help skills.

Now you can begin to see why Observational Early Intervention by you is so very important. The outcomes to the observations of your child's behaviours are the key to their support systems. No one else will know this stuff, you bring this vital information to the meetings, reviews, assessments, diagnosis and development chats, the IEP and EHCP meetings. You hold the key to the pathway that your child/adult/client will enter and how they see themselves for the rest of their lives.

I want to explain I am not suggesting you ignore a person if they are hurting themselves or others or breaking equipment—if harm is being caused there are times you will need to intervene. There are many ways this can be done—distraction with the right thing for that person can help massively. During observations you may learn what distractions you can offer to help break the momentum of any self-harming.

Just stopping the harmful behaviours isn't going to help at all. It may stop the harm the behaviour is causing but it will still leave a deep need to find regulation or feed the need that is there for such a behaviour in the first place. Remember, this isn't about bad behaviour where a child can be reprimanded, coaxed or negotiated with. We are talking about involuntary reactions to highly stressful/painful experiences affecting the whole person's experience. The important point is to replace it with another action that can soothe the incoming overloads or remove the harm/pain from the child's experience (loud noise) for example.

It is highly possible that by learning about the child/adult's sensory needs, the self-harm or harm to their environment or others around them will lessen or cease to exist at all.

Chapter 6
Finding Your Team

It is very beneficial to get a good team around you. Whatever your relationship is with the autistic person you are caring for or what your personal circumstances are, finding the right people and organisations can make a huge difference in helping you to positively support them.

If you are a professional, you know that team collaborations are usual—working in partnership with others is common practise and bringing individual knowledge to the table and sharing it creates a bigger picture in how a care package or support plan can benefit the person you are all working with.

I have found that when a positive relationship between professionals and parent/carers is established with the concept that all team members are equal, regardless of job title or status it creates a very constructive and beneficial outcome for the support and services that can be available to the child and family.

Having all parties consciously on an even playing field can mark out a mutual respect for each other's wisdom. A meeting of minds rather than a competitive mindset of who knows best or more.

Over the years I have heard of many situations where the parent/carer and the professional members feel defensive because they feel unheard, misunderstood and unsupported.

Sadly, this is currently happening in many schools across the Country and Globally. A breakdown of relations between the two wards. Parents/carers on one side the "professionals" on the other. Almost like a scene from a battlefield both armed and ready to defend their stance no matter what. This ends up in a complete breakdown of communication, nobody listening to the other. All the while the child needing support is left struggling.

The children and adults whom we are supporting reply on us to step up and advocate for them together.

Personally, I have experienced both disharmonious and harmonious relationships with teams of professionals. Guess which one had the richest impact for my son's needs?

Everyone involved in the latter felt heard, respected and valid. By putting our heads and hearts together with an attitude of equality, meetings were no longer stressful and fractured. So, I know it can be done and more so everyone feels better when it is accomplished.

If you are parenting as a sole carer, finding the right team for both you and your child is paramount. You may need two teams, one that assists you actively with the raising of your child, providing specific services in any areas they may require. The other are who support you in your parenting and personal needs.

If you are a parent/carer reading this, having time to yourself can be very beneficial. Space for you to relax and be free of decision making, planning activities or cooking, to name just a few. For some of you reading this, getting that space is difficult. I, too, over the years have had pockets of time with no adult company at all. I found ways of having my own space, which helped me keep my head above water. Your mental and emotional health is very important for you to find some way of decompressing and relaxing.

Over the years I have realised that support comes in many guises.

Obviously, we all need different things to help us feel relaxed and supported. You may find you have loads of small teams or groups of people who offer different elements. Siblings, Grandparents, friends, social media groups, supports workers, teachers, Social Workers, Speech (communication) therapists, Occupational therapists, nature, partners, even animals and pets can offer support and relief.

Hobbies too, or anything that gives you joy, may be a walk in the park bare foot, swimming for 30 minutes, jogging, dancing, singing, meditating, yoga…simply doing absolutely nothing! Definitely sleeping! Even a quick snooze can be amazingly helpful if your days are super busy. Whatever or whoever it is, that gives support to you is a team member.

Maybe it's someone listening to you rant, express your feelings of concern or overwhelm. Maybe you need a hug—no advice just a loving cuddle. Sharing the joys and celebrations of your child however big or small can also be such a wonderful boost.

Asking someone if they could grab some groceries for you can make a difference to your day, if your child struggles leaving the house and/or going to the supermarket—this is a huge help. We can also get a delivery much easier these days, I have opted for a food delivery so that when J is at school, I have more time to do other things.

Whatever our child's needs are, parenting is shared, although we may not recognise it as so, after all it is the parent/carer who has the ultimate responsibility to the child at the end of the day. BUT nevertheless, there are many other people in a child's life who contribute to their care and wellbeing, giving them a multitude of experiences to add to the essence of their lives.

Think of your own childhood, growing up you may have visited and had sleep overs at friends' houses, played in parks and mixed with others you met whilst out and about, never to be seen again. Maybe you attended dance or karate classes. Maybe you had study groups and other clubs that you attended regularly as well as spending time with family members, all of these people in essence helped raise you indirectly.

However, it isn't uncommon for the typical families and support groups (as above) to breakaway or collapse when a child cannot cope with everyday routines such as meeting for coffee at a park or going to the supermarket followed by a bite to eat in a café. Isolation is real when a child finds it tough doing transitions or has a routine based coping strategy. Sensory challenges can be the most difficult when you step outside the front door.

The reasons for this are varied and whatever the circumstances arc, when this happens, it can be extremely traumatic for you, the parent/carer which in turn can impact your child. If isolation slips into your life, it can become a constant reality. It takes courage and strength to ask for help and reach out to new groups.

Sometimes relationships breakdown because others struggle to understand the parenting choices you make and behavioural methods you implement. There are different views on how to "discipline" a child which can be a big divider between neurotypical and autistic child parenting.

Parenting advice is offered and everyone has their own view on how is best to deal with a specific situation. Often, though these different views will not match up to the reality and sensory needs your child has. Even the most well-meaning advice can be totally wrong for your autistic child, when there is high emotion, fear and tiredness mixed up with worrying about doing the "right" thing, sadly relationships can become challenged.

Some family members find it hard to accept a diagnosis, others may find it difficult to see a loved one (you) upset and feel the need to step in and "help".

For others, it is a different mindset, preferring to use historical behavioural methods that they feel worked for them as a child or with their own children. Usually this is due to a lack of understanding of your child's behaviours or simply not accepting they are autistic. This can add a huge dollop of pressure on you, trying to get others, especially family, to understand why your autistic child needs things done in a particular way that is completely different to how they raised you or were raised themselves.

Whilst these can be resolved in time, an incredible amount of patience is required of you on top of all the other worry you may have.

This can take a lot of your energy at a time when you are already stretched with your own emotions. Each family is different and knowing when to step back and when to ask for help is something you learn along the way. Asking family to read information or attend support groups can really help bridge the gaps of any misunderstandings, giving them this book to read may help too!

Speaking from your heart about your feelings and how they can help support you can be all that is needed. Sometimes, though it is simply too much to try and explain your feelings—the tiredness is alike to having a new born when sleep patterns are interrupted for a few months.

This is why I suggest speaking from the heart about how you really feel, trying to stay strong will prevent others from knowing just how lonely or tired you are. This takes courage, showing our vulnerability feels scary, I know I struggled and still do sometimes to let your self be seen as needing support. Yet at the same time, when I have allowed myself to do so—someone answers my call for help, one way or the other.

Emotional stress can fragment one's ability to ask for help, when that is the very thing, we need. It's a catch 22 situation. I have learnt this and it can be incredibly difficult to pull yourself from feeling wretched to then being able to admit you are needing emotional support.

I needed validation of my experiences and how I felt about them, not necessarily solutions to specific situations. Being heard, for me made a huge difference, it also helped me get stuff out of my head, which would often swirl around without me being able to stop it. Hearing myself speak it out loud helped me to release some of the pent-up frustrations and worry. I also learnt to not presume others knew what I needed, sometimes I would feel so tired with worry and overwhelm that to me it was obvious, of course no one knows unless you tell them. Years ago, I would find it difficult to share my feelings because I felt guilty. None of how I felt was aimed at my son, this was all my stuff. Yet by telling others, I worried that they would see my son in a negative light and I didn't want that. These feelings were what I went through in the early stages of being a parent. Years later to here and now, I have let all of that go. Mostly because I have found great friends and support both personally and professionally as well as allowing myself the grace to feel whatever it is I am feeling free of guilt.

Asking for help is definitely a skill and I strongly recommend you practise it as soon as you can. Having an autistic child has its tough lanes and it also has its wonderful ones. I do not mean because of your child, more so the meetings, phone calls, paperwork and assessments that are required to get a diagnosis and funding for financial support. On top of that is the social and educational structures we currently live in. I found that the appointments, expectations of attending them (when my son had huge difficulties leaving the house and entering buildings, especially waiting for ages to be seen), all of this created huge anxieties for me, worrying if we would be able to receive the support my son was entitled to because of the limiting methods of appointments. Since the pandemic appointments have become more creative, telephone and zoom are being encouraged which can make everything so much easier. Oh, how I wished that was an option when J was younger!

Some of your child's behaviours and struggles can be super difficult to cope with at first, especially when you have yet to learn why they may be upset and why they are behaving in certain ways. It is OK to say you are struggling, truth is every parent/care giver does when parenting/caring/supporting children. If it was all super easy, there wouldn't be support groups and forums to share worries and concerns.

This is where using social media platforms can be very positive. Groups that are connected with autism and neurodiversity are growing in numbers creating ample choice, therefore finding a group that fits your needs is completely possible.

Autistic/Neurodiverse led groups will be your saving grace, from the get go, you can ask questions and if they cannot help, you will be led to other groups for all manner of needs and any questions you have. More so you can introduce your child to groups that are run by other autistic children and young adults so that they can form friendships and share their joys and worries, forming friendships they may not have been able to have in the school classroom (for example)

I found that joining a variety of groups helped me in different ways. A mixture of autistic led groups is a key factor in positive support. It teaches so much about a neurodivergent brain. As a neurotypical person you will find conversing with autistic people and other Neurodivergent adults very different from neurotypical chat. This in itself is an education. It helps you understand your own child's communication processes.

You will learn that processing words and sounds can have a very different method and pathway to what you as a neurotypical person experiences. There is no way of you knowing these things unless you talk to other autistic people.

Of course, there are differences, that's the point, isn't it? A neurotypical brain is different to an autistic one. The key is to accept that and be OK with it. Celebrate the differences (not necessarily meaning jumping for joy and getting the bunting out) or may be so! I mean celebrate the fact that you accept the differences and find ways to help both you and your child communicate.

Once you find the groups that best suit and you begin conversing with individuals you will see that your child being autistic and different to the majority of children you know (statistically I mean) will no longer seem as severe. Now all the people you meet will have autistic children and/or be autistic or Neurodivergent themselves.

The good news is there are thousands of members in the multitude of social media groups all over the world. They are a mixture of amazing people who bring golden nuggets of wisdom and experiences that you may never get to read in a book or be told by a neurotypical person, no matter how many years' experiences they have had. I do not say this to be disrespectful, the truth is autistic people will know and understand far more about being autistic than someone who isn't! BUT this doesn't mean a neurotypical person cannot support your family—I have met many who are a wonderful positive support who spend time listening and learning from other autistic people.

There are now (thanks to the autistic communities) more neurotypical people and professionals who are mindful and knowledgeable of what autistic people need which is slowly changing systems and attitudes in many areas of support.

Psychologically this is super healthy for you, therefore it will be just as healthy and beneficial and crucial to your child as you will be conversing with their own communities.

Sometimes just sitting back and being an observer when first joining autistic led groups is extremely helpful. You can read through mountains of previously discussed topics at your pace on things such as therapies, appropriate language to use when addressing autistic people, toileting support, communication tools, if you have a question, you can guarantee someone else has already asked it—so you will find answers pretty quickly.

Through the thoughtfulness of the group's admin, articles written by autistic members, books and other resources are all saved for anyone to access and educate themselves on.

There are 100s of groups on social media for women, boys, girls, men, the LBGTQI+, non-speaking autistic folk from all around the world that you will find best suits you and /or your child/adult.

Finding, what I like to call "a soul family" made up of non-blood relatives elsewhere is so important. Feeling alone is no joke and thank fully no one has to be. I found that as I started to go to support groups and my son started school, I levitated towards like-minded people. Some were parents to autistic children; others were people who were interested in the same things as me. At that time, there were not many social media autistics led groups around, unlike now.

The face book groups (to name just one) are brimming with members who have daily posts and questions and advice on anything you could possibly think of. You will find nuggets of information that can ease your parenting/carers or professional relationships. You will definitely find useful help on all things legal regarding schooling and inclusion which could be very helpful to you.

Remember you can start your own groups up, generations of parents and carers before us did not have this gift of information and life experience from other autistic people. Using social media as a positive support network for yourself and family members is like a lifeline.

Getting a professional team to support you is also a good idea. This can take time but is definitely worth it. When it comes to needing extra support and attaining funding, this team can be of great benefit. The key to getting a good support team is knowing your child well.

Understanding their sensory needs confidently because you have spent time (early intervention) observing them through the eyes of sensory interaction and processing. Learning as much about them as early as you can means you can choose the right fit in social workers or Occupational therapists. (For example)

You are and will continue to be an equal member of that team. There really is no divide, no matter what you may have initially thought before you had your autistic child. You may feel at times you know nothing, but if you observe your child the way I am speaking of throughout this book, you will be bringing that knowledge to the table. Others will bring their own wisdom that you too will need, altogether creating a specialist team unique for the individual needs of your child.

I do want to reiterate this point because many of you reading this may not have had any childcare training or studying prior to becoming parents.

This can seem like a disadvantage when meeting with professionals of whom some may carry the label of autism expert or specialist. Although in some cases this may be true (if they are autistic themselves for example), they will not be experts with your child whom they have never met. All teachers learn from their students throughout their careers. If adults allow them to, it is the children who teach us who they are. Our job is to simply listen with all of ourselves and not just our ears.

Everyone within your new team will speak slightly different languages with dialects that vary. BUT the aim is the same, to give your child the best opportunities that support their individual needs throughout their lives, whatever setting they are in. As they grow and move through nursery and school so will the team of professionals, you though will be the one constant, the anchor.

Of course, you will learn new ideas and concepts from each other along the way. You though as the main carer will be the encyclopaedia of your child giving reference to a variety of areas that they need supported. Their job will be to provide that in a variety of ways.

You will be the reminder that not all autistic children are the same and not all therapies will work for all autistic children. Remaining focused on your child and their individuality is important.

It is easy to get swallowed up and become a part of the stereotype of what autistic children need. Stay strong and committed to the knowledge your child has given to you. Be open to new ideas and strategies remembering that you are allowed to stop or change anything if it doesn't feel right or your child isn't happy.

There is a great deal of urgency around currently about early intervention. This has become quite controversial over recent years. At first, this concept was deemed a brilliant idea and in essence it is.

BUT the thing to be mindful of is, why? What is the reasoning behind certain early intervention suggestions? Ask yourself the question in each area of topic discussed during the meetings. This is the kind of thing that gets discussed at the many meetings you can request or are invited to. This does not mean that every suggestion for early intervention is a bad one. I am inviting you to check in with all that you have learnt about your child so far (or will have done) before you make a decision. Its OK to say no to suggestions just as it is to say yes and you can change your mind at any time too.

The point of support is to enable your child to thrive as they are, not to try and create a neurotypical human. Obviously, this will be damaging to your child and as you continue to read this book you will see exactly why.

I mention this in this chapter because much of what your professional teams will be discussing are supports that can assist your child in all areas of their development, it is the whole point of such teams.

Of course, we all want our children to be accepted and part of the meetings and discussions will be you ensuring that happens.

When a child attending school uses a wheelchair, it is not expected or accepted to see in the ILP or the EIP or their EHCP (individual learning plan, Education individual plan, Education, health and care plan) stated they have to learn to get around without it. (For example) the autistic child is no different—if (for example) they need to have a specific soft toy or object carried around with them at all times, it needs to be included in their IEP and any other legal documentation as a requirement for their needs.

You do not need to apologise that your child's individual needs are complex and need accommodations to be put in place in order for them to feel safe and happy. By accommodations, I mean changes made by the teachers around the environment that can support your child's life in every way.

Commonly the emphasis is on the autistic person to make all the changes in their behaviours. Yet it is mostly the environments that need to be changed in some way to reduce any sensory overwhelm. In further chapters, I will talk about this in detail in regards to each of the senses to help you see how these changes create a happier environment for your child.

If you are a new parent/carer, all of this can feel completely overwhelming and exhausting. Take one step at a time and feel into what you need right now, making a list of priority can help get the whirring thoughts and worries out of your head. Finding the support you need to be able to function as positively as possible is key. Your child needs you to feel well and happy, and if that means receiving help from professional agencies such as social workers, counsellors or daily support for outings and activities that your child can attend whilst you rest, so be it.

You are not alone in this, please know this and trust that when you ask for help you can receive it.

Chapter 7
An Introduction to the Senses and Autism

Imagine being shouted at right in your face, having a multitude of objects rammed right in your eye view, have intense smells put right inside your nostrils at the same time have a load of people touch and scratch you and hold you down all at once?

Imagine your ears popping and hurting so much it causes you to prefer to head bang than deal with the intense sounds in your ears because it vibrates right inside of your body creating feelings of anxiety and nausea.

Imagine how it feels to hear, see, smell and taste sensations in your own home that cause such intense discomfort and overwhelm that you need to scream and hit yourself to try to filter out the sensory input attacking your internal and external systems. Add on top of that the inability to speak vocally and even if you could—you were too young to understand what is happening and so overwhelming is the experience you cannot find the space in your brain to tell anyone what is happening.

Well for many autistic children their daily experiences can FEEL just like that is happening to them.

Here we are at the part of the book where I will be talking about the sensory systems; all 8 of them. I will talk about each one in its individuality and how it can affect your child's daily life. This will include some examples in play and toys, food and eating choices as well as communication and self-help skills such as toileting and sleep related needs. There is so much to learn about the senses which is why I have broken them down.

Right from the moment we are born we are receiving and processing information using our sensory systems. During this neonatal stage in our physical experience, we are more like spectators or so it seems, who knows what we are actually seeing and experiencing at this early stage in physical form.

From my understanding, our senses are interacting with our environments, both externally and internally, however we are not yet developmentally aware of what they are from a cognitive perspective. Although the first year of our new lives are a rapid learning, quickly beginning to interact and explore our environment in a relational way, explaining what our senses are doing in regard to any pain, discomfort or pleasure is limited as a baby. Unless the carer is either physic or autistic themselves and even that can have its limitations with baby language and expression interpretation.

Obviously, this can vary from baby to baby but as we grow into the coming early months our awareness becomes more so, as we acclimatise to our physical environment. Although in those very early months we are unable to express most of what that feels like, the sensory systems in our bodies are very much receiving information.

As new parents caring for our babies taking them out in the fresh air for walks or in the car or bus they are drenched in a multitude of different voices, visual experiences, textures and temperatures. Food and drink and all the sensory flavours they bring of smell, sound, taste and touch. We can often miss the importance of the sensory experiences and take them for granted, not realising how they aid or hinder our baby's learning awareness, experiences and development.

Many years ago, during one of my jobs I met a young girl, aged almost 3 years old. She taught me a great deal about the need to experience all of what I have mentioned in the above paragraph. She was taken from her maternal home due to extreme abuse. Part of that experience for her was being deprived of those natural sensory experiences. She had never been outside in the fresh air, only knowing the small space of her parents flat. The curtains were drawn so sunlight and feeling the breeze on her skin didn't happen for her. She had never heard a bumblebee or a bird singing or felt or smelt the rain. She was given nothing to play with or experience herself with other than a darkened room and physical pain.

Part of my role was to help her become comfortable in her surroundings, especially the outside world. She taught me how important and necessary it is for a tiny baby to experience all of those natural elements which feeds through our sensory systems. She would scream when the wind blew, even gently, she would squint her eyes when outside as the day light was so strange to her. Being almost 3 she had a lot to catch up on and it took time.

Although it may seem that our tiny babies are not taking any notice of the elements and sounds around them, they most definitely do, meeting this incredible little girl taught me why it is important on a level I had never given any thought to previously.

The reason I have included this story is to reinforce the impact the sensory aspects of our living experience have, as well as being overwhelmed by them we can be under whelmed too. Her experience was extreme and helping her through those months and her learning what those invisible sensory experiences were was an education and an honour all at once.

We were teaching each other so much. A tiny scared 3-year-old taught me things no textbook could ever have done. She showed me how she felt and why whilst I stood by her side and followed her lead—gently guiding at her pace until she felt safe and able to cope.

As parents/carers we use our intuition to support our babies' needs and learn (eventually) what each cry sound means and what their body language is telling us. Some of it is luck (let's be honest here!) some of it is like a sixth sensory link we have with our babies. For that short time in our babies' lives we all learn how to non-verbally communicate. We accept our babies do not use spoken words and simply get on with it. We are relaxed as parents at this stage of their development and are happy to figure out and communicate in all the ways I have mentioned.

As our babies develop into their first year and often a little before, sensory difficulties can start to become apparent to the neurotypical eye…This does not mean they were not there before, rather they were not yet acknowledged and processed by baby, just as they were not recognised by the carer/parent.

From being inside the womb to then becoming a physical being, processing the intensity of the outside reality can take time to sort itself out and be realised. A bit like a flower coming into bloom. It is always a flower except whilst it is still within its bud and beginning to bloom it is not aware of the bees and the skies above it, being too busy with growing and adjusting to life itself.

It is often said by neurotypical parents when they reflect on their autistic child's development that it seemed the unusual behaviours came out of nowhere. How loud noises had never bothered their babies (for example) or their clothes were never an issue then one day they noticed their 12-month-old pulling at its clothes. This may be because a younger baby did not yet have the gross motor skills or coordination to be able to physically relieve themselves of such discomfort. Or they were, like the blooming bud and instead all energies were focused on adjusting to existing outside the womb. Or they were communicating their discomfort by crying or shutting down and sleeping a lot to deal with it but all of this got missed by the parent because it was deemed as "typical" baby behaviour.

I have found that more often than not it is thought that an autistic child's sensory challenges suddenly happen at around 12–18 months old (roughly). This was certainly the case with my son. I rewatched some family home video footage from new-born to his then current age. I was surprised to see that he was not responding to his name or my voice from as young as 8 months old, only occasionally which was enough to keep me from realising that he was autistic. (Obviously this was not the only thing that got me thinking he was autistic.) So, while I was living that moment with him, I didn't notice any of the behaviours that indicated he was autistic because I accepted them as typical baby behaviours that might have meant he was hungry, having wind or needing a cuddle. (Also, because sometimes that is exactly what he was telling me)

It is possible that any sensory overload (for example) that was being experienced by the young baby was completely missed. The parent has no way of knowing unless they have had previous experience of autistic sensory experiences or are autistic themselves. (That is if they know they are actually autistic, yet even being autistic yourself does not automatically mean you will recognise every behaviour and expression for what the truth of that it is) It's a guessing game.

When a baby cries, we all accept it as one of our main communicators of needing something. We are taught that it usually means that food or milk is needed or sleep, a nappy change or a hug and possibly some movement to help ease their stress.

I can bet the last thing most parents think of is that their senses are being overwhelmed. Even though typically for about the first few months it is common knowledge and practise to keep a baby wrapped up tight, maintain a calm and tranquil environment and rock or sway them to sleep. This could actually also be soothing any sensory needs your autistic baby has. Completely unaware though are the parents that it is sensory rather than just soothing to keep baby calm.

Around about the 3-month age, expectations change and the baby is thrown into a multi-sensory world of an epic scale—communication changes, voices get louder when speaking with baby, we clap and sing at close range. An array of baby rattles and sound making objects are shown and thrust into their tiny hands or up close in their faces, all to get a reaction to create a form of communication.

The point I am making is; a baby's way is to flap their hands and look sideways at stimuli, to smile or stare at what may look like nothing. Babies move their hands and wave their fingers in front of themselves and no one bats an eyelid or has any cause for concern. This is "typical" baby developmental behaviour. Just as it is typical baby behaviour to rock back and forth making repetitive sounds.

As we continue to grow and develop the neurotypical child's processing and sensory systems adjust and begin to filter out what cannot be handled all at once. The difference is that for the autistic sensory sensitive child this does not happen. Instead, the volume button of outside stimuli stays on high or it can become very low and unresponsive. This is usually when we (parents/carers) begin to see our children's behaviours becoming distressed, repetitious or unresponsive.

This too is the case in toileting and eating. It is accepted that a newborn baby cannot yet manage their own toileting needs. Then at a certain age (usually around 2-ish), the expectation is the child will begin toilet "training" the truth though could be that your autistic child has interoception sensory challenges right from birth, not being able to feel when they need to wee or poo was always there, how would a parent/carer know this? They wouldn't, it all starts to become apparent when the baby hits common milestone developmental stages.

This of course can look different for each child experiencing external stimuli when those systems have no filter management. Our bodies are always trying to help us stay safe, feel good or tell us something is bad by responding quite severely to certain incoming or internal sensory pathways.

This is why it can be difficult for a neurotypical person to identify or understand what this can feel like for the autistic person. It can be so extreme and overwhelming that behaviours created can look scary and even seem and be destructible or harmful to themselves and others.

For example, some behaviours can be screaming, headbanging, hitting oneself or others, scratching, laughing, flapping, spinning, vomiting, banging self or objects including other people. Eating all kinds of non-food stuff, chewing themselves or objects. Running around, jumping, not being able to sleep or sleeping excessively not responding to their name or other noises, or holding their ears to block out sound, even low sounds, sometimes movement alone can be too much to bear, laying on the ground, maybe screaming when being undressed or dressed, washed or showered, even hugged. This is a very short list of examples; the list can go on and be different for the individual.

Further on in chapters I will continue to list as many possible behaviours (communications) to help you understand the extent of sensory intensity and underwhelm.

Another factor making it difficult for a parent/carer to miss subtle challenges for their baby is their lack of knowledge of child development. Unless you have studied this for a career, it is unlikely that anyone would know this stuff. So be gentle with yourself for not always knowing what your baby, young child is feeling, needing or communicating.

I had this knowledge through my training in becoming an Early Years Professional. Studying all areas of child development from birth to 8 years old in detail. While this can be useful as the child grows, you can already see that during those new-born stages it didn't help me notice that my son was autistic straight away. Remember I had no knowledge of autism at all. The very nature of a new-born and its limited physical abilities means crying and sleeping or lack of is pretty much all they can do to communicate their distress.

More often, sleeping isn't seen as a sign of distress, although it most definitely could be a way of the baby shutting down any overwhelming sensory input. A bit like a coping mechanism that the body automatically does to protect itself. I am talking about over the average amount a baby sleeps. This was definitely one of my very early strategies. I slept all of the time and it certainly was and still is my son's.

Obviously, there are other reasons a baby may excessively sleep but on the subject of sensory processing and challenges—it can be a legitimate communication and coping solution of experiencing sensory overwhelm. We usually sleep when we do not feel well, our bodies shut down so that we can process and heal. We do this for physical, mental and emotional reasons, I didn't think about this being a possibility until I learnt about autism and its sensitivities, including meltdowns and shutdowns.

Now this makes perfect sense as an actual communication from the baby that they may be unable to cope with some sensory aspects of their being. I, myself slept excessively as a baby, much more than my 3 siblings, for me this was right from birth.

A lack of sleep for the baby can also be a communication of sensory overload, not being able to shut down enough to rest. Being so sensitive that they hear and sense so much it deters them from falling into a deep sleep. Most parents would not know that a musical mobile (for example) might not be soothing but instead the opposite, preventing the baby to relax and gently fall asleep. Others need very loud (what might seem inappropriate) for a young baby's ears, like drumming or brass band music, yes, really.

The majority of autistic adults know that they were born autistic. They didn't suddenly become autistic through other means or reasons. This is a huge subject and there are many discussions, theories, investigations and studies into what causes autism.

This book isn't going to get into those areas. (My point in mentioning this is perhaps all that is missed through natural baby behaviours is why it is often believed an outside factor made a child autistic.) Instead, I will be focusing on how to help you support the sensory needs of your autistic child or a client you have.

My intention in the coming chapters is to tool you up with as many possibilities and reasons for behaviours that your child/autistic person may be showing you. Furthermore, you can become knowledgeable and confident to inform teachers and psychologists of how your child functions and why.

I will be showing you throughout this process that all behaviour is communication. This becomes more apparent when you have a non-speaking child. That said, if your child does use spoken language this does not mean they can explain their needs or experiences easily. This in itself can be a sensory issue as well as a developmental process or an executive functioning issue, to name but a few. So! There is a lot to explore and discuss.

I urge you to be mindful of your own sensory experiences. This book, I hope will enable you to spend some inner time to explore yourself intimately. Most of us spend little time exploring intently what we hear, see, taste, touch and smell both internally and externally. Doing so whilst reading this can help you further understand how sensory experiences can impact your child/client.

I know I had not always lent myself the gift of listening to what my body was telling me, especially regarding food and processing letters, words, numbers and sound and smell. It just felt like a huge problem and I was either seen as a picky, fussy eater or a slow learner, not very helpful, in fact emotionally it made me anxious and worried, I had toileting problems too. I became very self-aware of my "issues" which in turn created more anxiety and magnified the fears of eating and learning, neither of which I could do confidently for many years.

You could use this book as a self-awareness activity and maybe discover things about yourself you had not before realised. One of the most surprising aspects of my own self-discovery into sensory processing was how much I automatically shut out or skimmed through without allowing myself to fully enjoy the full essence of (for example), a smell or taste.

By slowing down and thinking about each sense, I was able to be enriched by my life experiences. This meant I received far more pleasure in some of the sensory aspects, and in others I learnt I had challenges. More importantly I learnt why I had challenges.

Of course, my biggest gift was being able to understand my son. Although I cannot fully experience things in the same way as him, I definitely have a richer understanding of his needs and it opened my mind to a different pathway of thinking and problem solving for and with him.

During our lives the majority of people we meet do not endure such intensity in sensory experiences, or at very least it isn't presumed that there are issues. Teaching in schools is geared towards a neuro typical brain with no sensory processing challenges, which may be the reason many children mask (hide) any challenges they have. This can lead to having the assumption that they are lacking in intellect, which is usually not the case.

We have become better educated and accepting of differences such as Dyslexia in school. There is still more that can be implemented in the way of support to give children, once they are diagnosed, but it has improved since I attended school. Hopefully the more sensory differences are talked about and understood the follow through of this will be that schools can better support the children who have sensory processing differences. Sometimes this has been interpreted as a learning or intellectual disability. When all that was needed was a few tiny changes to the environment for the child to learn. As well as a lot of acceptance in how a child needs to self-regulate during a class. This too will be discussed further along the book.

As you can see, sensory processing is a huge topic. It is about being human in every way from the tip of our heads to the tips of our toes! I am excited to be sharing with you the intricate aspects of our sensory systems. We all have these systems, the differences for our sensitive children are the extent of their senses and how highly or lowly tuned they are. You will learn from your child that these can change on a daily basis, through age and natural development as well as when poorly, overwhelmed or super relaxed.

Another important factor is that development and progress happen for autistic children too. It may take longer than the expected "typical" time frames and it may fluctuate. Comparing autistic children to neurotypical children and what they are doing and how they play is a waste of time. It creates anxiety and frustration, worry and a feeling of despair. The two brain types are uniquely different so comparing each of their progresses is a pointless exercise. With patience finding a pathway to your child's sensory needs is far healthier and successful in terms of seeing a child thrive and be able to show their full potential than anything else I have witnessed.

This does not mean that our children are less abled in learning anything, it means they learn differently and have interests in things that often neurotypical children do not. There is a lot of focus in the assessment world of what is usually known as "appropriate play" or "purposeful play", yet our children teach us that there is no such thing. This is a made-up concept or I see it as restriction into what a child should be doing at certain ages and development stages. When used as a rough guide, it can be helpful diagnosing some conditions. However, in terms of play itself, it is pointless and a narrow-minded observation into a child's intellectual and cognitive abilities. Putting rules on how play is supposed to look will of course make it look like a child is lacking in skills, whilst others are unnoticed or completely dismissed.

Play is an exploration of the body and mind and how it can work together to create experiences. It is also a learning of such an array of endless possibilities of concepts and discoveries. Seeing things differently or using a "toy" differently to what is seen as the "norm" or the "appropriate" use of such a toy creates new concepts and experiences necessary for our world to evolve. All new ideas came from stepping out of the lane of "normal". History can show us that many an inventor, innovator was deemed mad for coming up with new ideas. Yet once created they were hailed as genius and applauded and celebrated for their creativity.

My follow-on book will be all about play and the 8 senses as it is a huge subject.

A huge part of learning about your child and how they process the world as well as an insight into their minds is through observing how they play. Play is valid without a "toy" bought specifically for a purpose. Say for example you buy your 1–2-old toddler an activity centre, buttons and levers that create sounds, words, lights and colours. They will explore this toy by pressing the buttons and delight in its cause and effect. The parent may expect the child to learn colours and shapes, follow instructions amongst other skills and feel a sense of achievement for their young child when they do, all of which is completely acceptable. Think then of your 7 or even 15-year-old autistic child who continues to delight in the toy. Suddenly this isn't so cute, or acceptable. Now this is seen as babyish or that phrase, I have always found annoying, "inappropriate".

Maybe your autistic child is seeing and feeling so much more than you can, maybe the sounds are so joyful to them that they can do it over and over because why would you not if it gives you so much joy? Why stop? Maybe the guarantee of such sounds every time they press that button gives them reassurance and a sense of knowing where they are in that flow of the day? Maybe it helps them navigate the time and routines of each day. Maybe it has become part of a huge pattern to help them know when teatime is, it may even help prepare them for it or another activity coming up.

Another example of the rules of play can be a child playing with a broom and dustpan set…the expectation is that the child learns how to sweep up and collect dust etc. We celebrate our child's skills when this happens. Nothing wrong with that. Yet when another child holds the brush to their mouth or feels the bristles with their fingers or waves it around their bodies and shrills with delight everyone starts to panic. That's not how you are supposed to play with that!

Maybe the bristles feel amazing, the sound they create when touched feels so good and brings deep joy. Or the texture and weight of it in their hand helps them know where their own hands begin and end and they can feel their bodies in the space they are sat in?

This may sound strange but as you begin to look into sensory processing for a sensitive child you will begin to realise the purpose of all "play" it is a deeply personal experience when allowed to be. The rulebook can be thrown out, for parents and carers this can (and will be) extremely liberating. Plus, it helps to accept the many other different things your autistic child may do in public! It helps you develop a thicker skin when it comes to outsiders, strangers, even family members who may see things differently.

Of course, there will be many activities and experiences that both autistic and neurotypical children enjoy alongside each other and together. Those of you who have both neurotypes in your family will already be aware of this. There are no fixed rules here, instead opening our minds to all possibilities, seeing the goodness and the worth in all interactions.

Ok, let's get into the sensory categories and discover how your child explores their environment.

Chapter 8
Auditory Senses (Hearing, Sound)

Let's start with the sense of hearing, the auditory sensory input and output. This is an area my son has taught me so much in as he has auditory sensory sensitivities. I too have very sensitive sound input, nowhere near my son's but enough for it to cause me discomfort and other feelings I will explain as we go along in this chapter.

When my son was a baby (from around 12 months old), he began banging his head on the ground and walls. He would take himself off to quiet places, particularly where there were no other people. If we were out, say in a soft play centre where it is always noisy, he would be found under a tunnel or laying on the ground. He would enjoy the balls and slides, climbing and spinning on all its offerings but he would need to decompress throughout his time there and would always be the first child to want to leave. He could cope with this highly noisy, brightly lit busy place for no more than an hour, sometimes as little as 20 minutes. It wasn't unusual for it to take us up to an hour to get somewhere to spend just 20 minutes in the building to then return home.

At first, this was difficult for me to cope with. Feeling frustrated because of all the effort I had gone to in driving him there. My expectation was that he should enjoy being there for at least a couple of hours to make it "worthwhile" going in the first place.

This was very early days for me in my parenting journey and experience. It impacted more when I had arranged to meet other mums with their kids. They could sit and chat with coffee and food, while I was away with him ensuring he was OK and that he was safe. I too wanted to have the time to chat and eat and be that kind of parent, where we all meet up and let the kids run around playing for a few hours until they needed a drink or some food. I realised this was not going to be my experience as a parent. Until I did accept this my life seemed hard and frustrating, I constantly felt I was missing out on this "parenting experience" that everyone else appeared to be enjoying.

Once I changed my mindset, it all became easier. Jeorge (my son) was who he was wherever we went. It wasn't personal to me and while I continued battling with the idea that I was missing out on something, life seemed harder and I could feel myself falling down a rabbit hole of misery and self-woe is me. This didn't feel right either, because I wanted to learn about my son and help him enjoy his life experiences and it was my job to do so.

Bearing in mind he found it incredibly difficult to leave the house and enter any buildings, once I took myself from the mindset of me missing out, I began to see our trips out as successes when he could enjoy such a place, however long we were there for. I realised this was a stepping stone for his self-learning and life development of his sensory needs and challenges. Each year he could cope with longer visits, it just took a bit more time. I realised that my time with friends couldn't be during those situations, so I stopped trying to make it happen. This made a huge difference to my personal happiness, it had nothing to do with my son, more what my attitude and expectation to the situation was.

Auditory sensory processing affects every waking moment of life. We live on a planet where we create a lot of noise. There is no escaping it. Imagine being near a really high-pitched sound that you just cannot bear.

It makes you want to close your eyes and cover your ears and you may start to feel nauseous if kept there too long, giddiness can take over and your mind can become scrambled. A general feeling of stress and anxiety builds up until you just have to run, leave, get away from it as quickly as possible. If there is a build-up of noise for me, personally I can become giddy and hyperactive, sometimes I shake and need to shout or cry.

As soon as you are away you begin to feel better, balanced and calm. Generally, humans can cope with loud, even a multitude of sounds, pitches and tones automatically closing them off, easily without even thinking about it. For the auditory sensitive autistic, it simply doesn't happen that way.

Sitting in a busy café or pub is a great example. At first, typically we can hear the plates, cups, coffee machines and the many voices chattering away all at once. After a while, it all kind of fades into the background and you can happily sit, eat and chat to your friends for a pleasant time.

We all have certain tones, octaves of sound that we find unpleasant or joyful on a general human level. What we are talking about here is very different. This is an auditory system that is felt throughout the whole body. Like it enters and then explodes inside of you creating all manner of sensations and experiences. Sound isn't just a sound it becomes a complete physical experience. This can be pleasant beyond measure, blissful even, or it can be excruciating, overwhelmingly painful and all encompassing. It can create experiences where the whole body shuts down while trying to process or rid oneself of the experience that sound is causing. If I wear ear phones or headphones for too long, my ears swell up a bit, the vibration in them causes my ears to expel liquid and they throb.

Think about yourself for a moment, have you ever been to a noisy busy place such as a restaurant or pub, you felt healthy and vibrant and you had a fabulous time, not even giving it a second thought? Another time perhaps you felt particularly tired, or a bit hungry. You may have had a tough few days leaving you feeling stressed or worried about something. This day, suddenly the noise of the pub is disturbing, you find it irritating and your concentration is compromised.

What other feelings come up? Maybe you close your eyes to somehow help you feel some ease from the invasive stimuli? Maybe you tap your hand on the table or deep breath. Maybe you feel a little dizzy or sick, your heart beat or your temperature increases, causing you to shake a little? Or if overwhelming enough, you bolt, leave and get out of there as quickly as possible, feeling instantly better. Or maybe you feel a bit tired or energy drained, even a bit disorientated until you have had a bit of time to decompress from the overwhelm.

For many sensitive autistic children, this kind of experience (this is one example) can be an everyday and all-day reality. Thinking about it in these terms, you will realise how well your child does to exist on this planet with its many sounds (they are the ones you can hear, for there are many others that you typically cannot hear but the autistic auditory sensitive person can—and loudly)

Having auditory sensitivities and needing to shut out such overwhelm can be impossible, especially when younger. Entering a room or a building with that amount of noise will feel like torture. The noises can fill the body up from the inside, shaking every organ and bone. Their head may feel like it is going to explode creating intense feelings of fear and a need to get rid of it anyway they can.

The younger the child the less experiences they have had of anything, therefore noises are an enigma. Until they can build up their life experiences and match up what is making the noise, everything they hear will be non-relatable. All of this added together can create pain (emotional or physical) because of the actual noise and fear of the unknown.

Sometimes the noise of an activity or place can be the reason a child does not want to take part or enter. Not the activity itself. This can be a tricky one for a neurotypical parent/carer to figure out. For example, my son has always adored water, like it is his bliss place so we regularly took him swimming from a baby. During those baby stages he seemed unaffected by the noise of others or the echoes created by the huge building, voices and water, swimming instantly and breathing under the water with ease, eyes open and laughing it was incredible to witness.

As he got to around 12 months old things changed. We carried him into the poolside as we had previously done. This time he began screaming, as he threw himself on the ground his screams got louder. We thought he needed to leave so we tried to lead him away. No, he kicked and screamed more, squirming to get down. Confused we put him down yet he continued to scream and kick, laying by the side of the pool. He looked like he was in deep trauma which was difficult for me to watch and do nothing. People were beginning to stare and lifeguards were showing concern. The intensity built as the other swimmers were staring and whispering, wondering what on earth was going on. His screams echoed around the building and it looked like my son was having a horrendous time. We continued to see if he needed to leave but he refused instead lay back down alongside the pool.

This took a huge amount of trust on our part as his parents, instead of just ignoring his need to stay and continued screaming we could have scooped him up and removed him. We knew he loved water; he was always in it at home, either a bath or a paddling pool or in the ocean or a river. He had also shown us how he loved being in a swimming pool on past visits. So, instead, we trusted him and just like that, after around 30 minutes he jumped into the pool as happy as Larry! I recall him being in there for almost 2 hours.

Over the years this became less until eventually he learnt to self-regulate by closing off the input to sound by pressing with his fingers the bottom of his ear entrance. He still at 17, uses this method and continues to enjoy swimming, especially under the water, where of course it is quieter.

You see, he was teaching me that the activity itself was what he really wanted to do, the noise was the problem. He weighed up the need and want to be in the water, versus the crippling sounds around him. Even at 1 years old, he had the determination to endure that obvious discomfort so that he could get to his bliss place.

Here is a slightly off topic story but it does illiterate the above example with regards to a behaviour which may not always mean what you think it does:

Years ago, I met an autistic lady who was giving a talk, she explained her love of trampolines and her deep fear and loathing of dogs. YET the behaviour of seeing either of those things was exactly the same. For it was the intensity of the feeling both gave her, that created the same behaviour. This is something to be mindful of, it would be very difficult for someone to figure out especially if the behaviour is kicking and screaming.

Think of a situation or a place, a memory, music, maybe a movie or a person you loved (or not!) that leads you to tears, it can be a happy or sad experience it's the intensity that creates the same reaction. This is another part of the language you need to learn…Which isn't always easy.

Ok, back to the auditory sensory chapter!
Witnessing my son with new environments and the sounds around him is like he is tuning in a radio. Imagine when you are trying to find a radio station you enjoy, searching as you turn or press the button, all you can hear is distortion in between the stations. Then peace! You find your

desired station and it plays clear and the distortion goes. It's like he needed time to adjust to the frequencies of the pool and echoes of voices, screams and splashes as well as the lights and vast space. He could hear everything at once. Somewhere in him he had a place he could go where he could cope with the external sounds. He just needed time to find it, align with it and then he could enjoy the part he adored—the water.

He has shown me this throughout his life over and over again. Of course, we have bought him sound defenders to wear whenever he wants too. For some children, this will be their choice to do so. For Jeorge, he prefers to use his fingers to control the volume coming into his ears. Occasionally when at the cinema or theatre he will wear ear defenders, but only for short bursts of time. I think it is the pressure on his ears that cause him some discomfort whereas his fingers don't and this method is productive for him.

As I mentioned earlier, he would headbang throughout the day where ever we went, even at home. We realised that those early months and years of him doing so was his way of trying to deal with the auditory input, he was too young to figure out a strategy that wasn't harmful to him. The one that worked was to head bang or whack himself in the forehead. It got so bad and regular that he had a permanent lump and bruise, sometimes a cut across his forehead. Remembering back to those times, I would lay awake at night terrified he wouldn't wake up from a sleep, having a bleeding brain or severe concussion.

Along with a couple of other sensory needs he had (which I will be speaking of in other chapters) this was the reason he headbanged. So, what looks like a mindless behaviour was in fact a coping strategy for him, even as young as 1-year-old.

Auditory overwhelm can be caused by many aspects and things. It will be different for every autistic child/adult who has this particular sensitivity and be mindful that any examples or lists I give are not exhaustive, there will be many I have not listed. Instead, my aim is that the examples I give here will help you think in different terms and why they may be happening. Rather than seeing them as behaviours that are either "bad", "naughty", "unacceptable", "inappropriate"; instead understand and accepting that EVERY BEHAVIOUR HAS REAL LOGICAL MEANING TO THE PERSON COMMUNICATING AND EXPERIENCING IT.

If you learn what is causing your child to create behaviours that are dangerous or damaging to them or others, it can be crucial to helping them find solutions and alternatives. Many of your child's behaviours and responses from their environment will not be harmful, they may stand out and look odd but they are always an interaction and communication either with the experience itself or as a response to it, whether that is a noise, a smell, touch or a taste or an internal feeling of pain, body function such as needing the toilet or feeling hungry.

Your child is expressing themselves in their way, a valid language of their own that can be learnt by others if they are willing to listen and watch without the need to change or stop it.

For many of our autistic, sensitive children who are non-speaking— behaviours will be their words, which also expresses their emotions. Which is why learning this form of language and communication is vital.

Senses can overlap and intertwine with each other, after all we experience many things through our senses at once every second of the day. Separating them can become tricky. Hereon in I will endeavour to explain this.

My son can be affected through his auditory senses with lots of movement that isn't making any sound that is obvious to anyone else. I have learnt that my son can hear vibrations so acutely that a group of animals, say cows who are not creating any obvious sounds such as mooing can cause him to press his ears closed and deep breathe, close his eyes until he has passed them. This happens daily when we are passing them in the car, windows shut. He cannot hear them from their sounds but he can through their energy and vibrations. He still does this, although now he is a teenager. We live rurally so cows are a plenty. He does this with horses too and other animals.

This happens when watching documentaries on TV that are about animals. Mostly the big animals such as buffalo, wildebeest, lions, tigers and birds that are in huge flocks. I have experimented with the volume on the TV, the sight of them alone can cause the same reaction and need to close his ear opening. He does this too with mountains, vast oceans that we either drive past, through or he sees on TV. WHY? It could also be that he is anticipating the known sounds that these animals make.

I have learnt that it is also the vibrations he can hear. Many animals have super acute ear and can hear different sound waves and notes that humans cannot. Just because a sound is not heard by you, does not mean it isn't there. These animals can hear sounds from miles away, they can sense an approach from another animal way before a human would be able to.

For our auditory sensitive children/adults, this is true also. It is a scientific fact that everything vibrates, which creates a sound. Researching this is easy, there are many resources that show you the sound of tiny animals, insects, flowers or mountains and the sound they emit. Each human too has a unique sound, I am not talking about the sound of our voices that's something different. This is the sound we create when simply existing. Even mother earth has a sound of her own, planets all have sounds. I recommend you take a look at some websites; NASA have some great recordings of planetary sounds, the sun, moon and earth…

This is some text taken from a website search of 'everything in life is a vibration' that explains what I am speaking about:

'Flowers take on their shape because they are responding to some sound in nature. Crystals, plants, and human beings are music that has taken on visible form.'

Never underestimate the level of sensitivities your child may have. What you cannot hear, can be heard by your child in a real way. So, imagine a busy place, full of people—it may not be noisy in terms of talking but the mixture and number of people in one space will create a louder sound, than having one or two people in a space. Add on top any talking, walking sounds, the rustling of clothes, breathing, then add birds, traffic, machinery, music, cutlery the list goes on. Another layer is to then add tones, volume, pitch and suddenly what seems like a relatively quiet space to you can be a noise, an orchestra of sounds so loud shutting it down is necessary to feel safe and at ease. Here is a list of what some behaviours and overwhelm of sound can create;

Head banging
Scratching
Hitting themselves or others or something
stamping
Screaming
Laying on the ground
Running away
Laughing
Crying
Rocking
Spinning
Climbing
Sleeping
Hiding

Vomiting
Closing eyes
Shouting
Humming
Pinching

Here are a few activities that may be difficult to experience, some that you may not consider to be an auditory problem:

- Haircutting (loud noise of scissors)
- Hair washing/brushing
- Singing
- Talking (themselves and others)
- Shouting/screaming—words may become distorted so unable to understand what is being said
- Shoes on the ground
- Traffic
- Sirens
- Music, some instruments
- Scraping of chairs, tables
- Cutlery
- Eating/chewing/slurping/swallowing
- Lights humming
- Animals sounds (certain types)
- Sound of zips
- Doors banging
- Machinery
- Hoovers, mowers
- Kitchen appliances such as kettles, washing machines, mixers, coffee machines
- Electronic games
- Pouring of liquid

I have learnt that movement can cause my son auditory issues. I will explain, as an example, when he is sat in the car with the windows closed, he cannot hear (sound) or what is going on outside, yet he can "hear", feel something which causes him to close off the entrance to his ears. (Unlike the cows I used previously as an example) This could be the changing of pressure as we live in Wales and are often going up and down hills! It could be the anticipation of certain sounds or it could be the change in vibrations he can hear on the earth?

Visual sound is real too, I have experimented with the volume controls on the TV and even with the sound turned down he will act as if the sound is up when looking at mountains, vast oceans, trees, people, buildings, bridges, most things…he has always done this and continues to do so. He hears with such depth and intricacy he misses nothing. Which is impressive but it can and does cause him discomfort. Sometimes intensely where he will start to pant and deep breath to help counteract the affect it has on him. He closes his eyes too, sometimes he laughs loudly which can mean he is doing his best to cancel out the incoming sound/vibrations. (This can also be because of visual stimulation, more of this is explained in visual chapter.)

He can also find some sounds, notes, melodies, tones, patterns funny. Some musical instruments and how they are played and in what tunes etc. can cause him to laugh. During my relationship, closely observing him I have learnt to see why he finds such notes funny. I am listening differently, now somehow tapping into the language he is hearing and sometimes I giggle too, I get it.

This is one of my main realisations and one that I want to pass onto you. When we watch quietly our children's reactions and relationship with the sensory input and environment stimuli, we too enhance our senses. This helps us understand our children which means we can support them more easily and therefore help others such as teachers and family members to support our children too.

Our kids live in this world and while we cannot ask it to stop making all its noises, being unpredictable, busy and fast we can learn why our kids behave as they do and help them to find ways to live in the world without having to suffer so much. This is where my version of "early intervention" comes into play.

Now we have established that everything has a vibration it may not surprise you to hear that taste too can create a sound wave inside the body. Just as it can create other sensory reactions. We are also talking about synaesthesia which is a stand-alone condition that any human can have and not be autistic or have sensory processing challenges in any way.

'Synesthesia or synaesthesia is a perceptual phenomenon in which stimulation of one sensory or cognitive pathway leads to involuntary experiences in a second sensory or cognitive pathway. People who report a lifelong history of such experiences are known as synesthetes. (Taken from a google search heading.)

Some children and adults will be able to hear their food depending on the colour it is, or the size, the type of food it is…although these examples are less common, I felt it worth mentioning because it all adds to us learning about possibilities and understandings of our children's sensory sensitivities. Being autistic and sensory sensitive is a whole other level of interacting with the world, we can leave no stone unturned, however unfamiliar to you it may be.

Drinking and Eating

Auditory sensitivity can cause a lot of interference in food and eating. It's a noisy department! From buying it, packing it away, preparing and cooking it to then eating it. This can add to your child not wanting to eat or being cautious about where, how and what they can or want to eat.

(Remember my point about not liking the noise of an activity but really wanting to take part in the activity itself without the loud noises?)

It is a possibility that an auditory sensitive child might want to eat because they are hungry or really does like what is on offer, yet the noises of others eating or the scraping of chairs and cutlery on the plates, slurping of drinks, chewing, talking…all creates too much overwhelm and discomfort that they withdraw from eating at all. Whilst feeling very hungry and frustrated that they cannot take part.

Breaking every part down and individualising it can help you clearly see where your child will have difficulties.

If sound is something, your child is sensitive to, eating could be a challenge for them. Not only for the incoming sounds from cooking and others eating but also their own sounds when eating. Chewing, swallowing and crunching can be an incredibly loud internal experience, enough to cause some to eat as few times as possible.

This can be another of those examples that they may want to eat and feel hungry but the sensory issues are too much to cope with. My son finds eating crunchy food incredibly difficult, although he loves his toast in the morning (it is very lightly toasted as he will not eat it as untoasted bread) as part of his routine (ritual and routine are extremely important and vital for him) So he needs to eat his crunchy toast whilst making a loud vocal sound himself—this somehow helps balance out or even dim down the sound the crunching of his toast makes. He also claps whilst eating, he rubs his ears and sometimes closes his eyes. We avoid as many crunchy foods as possible, however the act of eating and chewing is naturally noisy internally. His clapping is loud, this enables him to eat and cope with the intense sensory experience. Stopping him from doing this whilst eating would be detrimental to his health and wellbeing. He would most likely, cease to eat at all. He spent 7 years eating only a handful of chips and 2 dry buns a day, now he eats a large variety of nourishing foods. So, the clapping and vocal sounds with the need to stand up whilst he eats are in fact an enabler for him to eat at all.

This is a prime example of changing the environment or circumstances/rules/expectations and not the person's actions/needs. Rather, accept the need for such actions and behaviours by understanding his sensory needs—I ensure that wherever Jeorge spends nights or days away from home they honour his requirements.

Environment can play a huge part in preventing a person from being able to or wanting to eat. Finding the right circumstances can make the difference in them being able to eat at all.

Usually, we are expected to eat with other people or worse still in restaurants, cafes and other busy places. I personally struggle with this, especially places with loud coffee machines and kitchen areas of crashing plates and cutlery.

If this is an area your child struggles with and they are auditory sensitive, this could be the reasons they do not eat with others or in the same room with people. (There could be many other reasons too) Such as hearing the chewing and slurping of people when eating can be invasive to their ears. For my son, it caused him to gag and wretch. When he was younger, he couldn't cope with seeing animals on the TV eating because of the noises they made. He found that impossible with us and other family members. So, we changed his environment which enabled him to eat peacefully.

We let go of any rules or expectations of needing him to sit with us to eat, more important was that he ate. So, he ate in a room on his own or with his favourite DVD on, whilst sitting down and standing up or even walking around—going back and forth to his plate to finger eat his meal.

Once we allow ourselves to get rid of social rule expectations and instead understand that it is not beneficial to tell our children (especially those who have severe sensory issues) how to eat their food. Most adults I know eat food in all manner of ways and places that could be seen as anti-social, yet it happens. Why, then do we expect so much from our children?

We can of course, encourage and suggest to our children to sit at a table, a chair or on their bottoms whilst they eat using utensils etc. If, however this is clearly a struggle for them and they show different methods in eating comfortably, why not follow their lead? Especially if you do not know how the child is feeling and what makes it so difficult for them to eat in the "so called socially acceptable way".

Here are a few examples of ways an auditory sensitive child may want to eat:

- Standing up to have ease of movement
- Stand up and sit down in short spurts
- Tapping their feet
- Jumping from one foot to the other
- Laughing loudly
- Making loud noises whilst chewing/clapping
- Stimming with their bodies or hands
- Moving around the room
- Having breaks during a meal (sometimes eating a meal can take all evening)
- Needing to engage with another activity such as an iPad
- Wearing ear defenders to help with the noise others make
- Eating only soft food—non-crunchy
- Eating only crunchy food
- Eating only round or triangle (any specific shape)
- Eating only one colour of food

- Eating foods that are only dry
- Eating the same foods at the same time each day
- Eating specific food on specific days sometimes in adherence to a particular activity that happened that day
- Eating food that does not touch another on the plate
- Eating foods in a particular order
- Eating only one particular brand of food
- Using fingers and hands to eat instead of cutlery as it creates a sound on the plate and may feel horrible in the mouth
- Using a straw to drink with to avoid slurping and huge swallowing actions

Most of the above examples are deemed anti-social in the meal time "unwritten rules" yet the difference they can make to a child being able to eat happily without stress is incredible.

Eating under stress has very real emotional effects on a child creating big issues around food and drink for many years to come. It can also create digestive health related issues such as acid reflux, vomiting, indigestion and ulcers; to name a few.

Often things can change in time, as your young child develops and becomes more experienced within themselves. Having their needs met can help them become stronger and more able to cope with issues they could not previously. Remember everything is a stepping stone to something else. I have learnt this as a very valuable factor in my son's life and development. It is so worth taking the time and doing things the way they need it done, however that looks to anybody else.

Out and About in Shops and Other Social Places

Supermarkets are an auditory sensitive person's nightmare—sound, movement, colour, people, trolleys, all create a barrage of tones, pitches and volume which is chaotic and incredibly LOUD.

The sheer size of a supermarket generally can create such a loud sound of echo and feedback that entering one is incredibly distressing. This is a place my son will still not enter. Because I understand his sensitivities, I accept this. Instead, I shop either online (which I personally prefer and get it delivered) or I go when he is at school, now he is older I leave him in the car if I need to pop in and grab a few things. For some of you, this is difficult if you have no babysitters or family members to watch your children. I urge you though, if you can avoid your child having to endure a supermarket if they find it stressful, then do.

Remember the stepping stones I mentioned earlier? There is plenty of time to help your young child with entering buildings such as supermarkets. Although these days it isn't necessary when online shopping is available from all supermarkets, even to collect it whilst sat in your car.

There are some strategies used and suggested by some professionals and therapists (especially behavioural) that involve desensitising your child by exposing them to experiences that cause them distress, in short bursts. The idea is that eventually they will "get used" to it and not "behave" in that way anymore. The validation of this method stems from the attitude of "they have to learn to live in the real world".

The first point to remember is your child is in the real world as an autistic person, experiencing it in a very close up and magnified way, yes, it's very real! I am sure you would agree that having to live in constant despair is not a necessary part of living in the real world.

The other point is that desensitising can create bigger problems for your child that may become internalised. This can be immediately or as time goes by. Anxiety and mental illness can increase and a serious lack of self-judgement.

This can create huge trust issues of others and even worse they will not know how to trust their own instincts when it comes to dangerous situations. Using such severe methods as desensitising so abruptly can have a counterproductive effect. Whilst it may look like certain behaviours are being stopped or controlled, what is happening instead could be an internalisation of needs and fears.

Behaving in ways that please others and compromising their own, is known as masking—a form of suffering in silence and living a miserable life. The truth is that usually as the young child ages and has more time to learn about themselves they slowly build up their experiences on their own terms. Things can become slightly easier for them in many areas of life.

My son can go into a few buildings, but it has taken years of patience and acceptance. Loads of preparation, explanation, choices, a B plan and more patience. Compromise and sometimes even letting go of an idea completely. There are other reasons he cannot cope with large buildings but sound and noise are the main factors.

Play and Interaction with Others

Play can be a noisy affair and being around other children is too. Unpredictable noises, screams, cries, laughter, voices; not to mention the noise of the toys and equipment. When you look at it from an auditory sensitive perspective, playing and being on your own isn't a lonely place—it's heavenly!

This could be a factor as to why your child finds engaging with you or others through play difficult. (I remind you that there may be other reasons too) for this aspect of the sensory realm, sound is a huge factor.

Most toddler toys are noisy…We (society) have a need to overload our kids with sounds of every type. Music, beeps, banging, clapping, animals, voices—it's endless. So, for an auditory sensitive child this is trauma inducing. Suddenly playing on your own or finding a cupboard or an outlet of some kind will be much more welcoming than needing to interact with peers. What looks like loneliness to you could be joy/peace/bliss/less painful or distressing for your child.

It may be surprising to hear that although my son is extremely sound sensitive, he also seeks sound and enjoys listening to a variety of them. BUT, BUT, BUT only when he has control over those sounds, experienced on his own terms. It is like he is trying to overcome his discomfort by listening to sounds through a variety of means, as well as figuring out the intricacies of each sound.

Let me explain…

He loves classical music, we found out when we used to watch a classical music video channel. He would stand close to the TV and listen, the TV was on low and he loved the sound of the music and the melodies, he would show a deeply connected emotion of appreciation too. He began showing a big interest in sound books, the kind that has sound buttons down the side of the book or have buttons to press throughout a story. He still has many scattered around our lounge which he listens to every day as part of his routine. He has one finger pressed against one ear entrance and experiments with the volume control of this. He has around 50 of these books now. From animal sounds to favourite character story sounds such as Peppa pig or Gruffalo's child, machinery, car, lorries, sea life, birds, dinosaurs the list is vast. The difference here is he can manage these sounds; they are not forced onto him.

He enjoys the sounds of many things. Yet he finds them overwhelming when he cannot monitor where and when they arrive at his ears. By being mindful of his auditory needs and challenges when he was younger to the point of avoidance has enabled him to become aligned with sounds in a natural way. Being human, we cannot avoid having any of our senses closeted. What we can do as parents and carers to our sensitive children is slow down and manage their environments as much as possible so that life for them is less stressful, traumatic and scary.

Eventually, as they grow and learn how to manage their sensory needs themselves you can help them explore the world more openly. Rushing this process can be counteractive instead creating severe stress and anxiety and a less want to interact with anyone or activities, they may have come to enjoy given time.

Throughout this chapter you have learnt that one sense overlaps/ affects another (obviously we use all our senses at once). This can multiply an autistic person's experience in everyday life. Depending on the autistic persons personal sensory system this can be intense and overwhelming—it is easier, then to look at an autistic person's behaviours that were once seen as confusing or unusual to in fact having logic and reasoning, seeing them now as a communication, a language of interaction or as a reaction to the environment or experience at that time.

This is a huge subject; I recommend more research into them or to engage in further self-discovery. This first book, is an introduction to the senses and autism combined, giving you a condensed idea of what each sense is and how it can affect an extremely sensitive system.

Sound to Cover Other Sounds

It isn't unusual to see an auditory sensitive child/adult creating sounds themselves constantly. Humming and clicking, singing, shouting and many other sounds are created to sometimes drown out other more painful or unpleasant sounds they are experiencing.

You can also be sound sensitive and sound seeking—the latter needing lots of noisy loud banging and such like. Hearing the sound of crashing toys down the stairs or across a floor. Banging on doors or floors to name a few. (This could be for other sensory reasons too.)

All of this can be figured out by you, the carer when you observe your child as much as possible. Once you have learnt what it is your child is experiencing (to the best of your ability), you can then assist the environment to relax most of the external sounds (or increase noise of certain types if they are seeking sound), creating a more peaceful and easy existence.

Obviously, you cannot make the world quiet, but you can certainly help in many ways. When someone is suffering all day every day, enough to create extreme behaviours I have mentioned—easing this in any way you can becomes easy and natural.

Imagine having to exist with a constant extremely loud radio on in your ears all the time? (An example) Eventually you wouldn't be able to function. If you were expected to put up with it, you would start to behave in a way that may look weird or extreme to others. When all you are trying to do is find a way of filtering out such extreme noise.

Headphones/ear defenders are an obvious strategy, some though can be difficult to wear, putting pressure onto the head or ears. They can make people feel giddy or afraid, because they can block out too much sound and cause issues with the vestibular sensory system, which is another chapter further along. If there are touch sensitivities' wearing ear defenders can be impossible. Each year there are new types of noise-cancelling equipment on the market, I will be trying some new loop type ones for my son this year.

Music may help while wearing earplugs, there are many available these days that sit outside the ear. (If the person can tolerate them on).

The most important point is that you accept any type of stimming that will help filter or cancel out the extreme noises that may be causing problems for them. If they are harmful to the person, this means obvious damage to their bodies or others then finding another way to help filter out excess sounds and suffering is possible, it may take time but it is possible.

Remember sometimes with sensory support more stimulation to that sense might be needed, loud sounds, pitches, tones, beats, words, particular musical instruments—some may seem unpleasant to you but calming and satisfying to the person with the sensory issues.

Finding out the intricacies of what your child is experiencing and what and why they need adjustments takes time and careful observation. You may make mistakes numerous times, needing to play around until you both can find the solutions.

Remember as your child grows and develops, their needs will too—they will find their own strategies more easily and as you learn about them you will see more clearly the strategies they are already using. Everything becomes clearer when you learn their sensory language through their behaviours.

Chapter 9
Touch/Tactile

Touch is unavoidable in human existence, from the moment we are born we are touched and held, whether that be skin on skin or clothing along with a vast variety of materials.

Many humans thrive on touch, it is a pleasurable and joyous form of human expression and deep need to feel loved and safe. For skin/touch sensitive people, the opposite is real, yet the need to be held, hugged, squeezed in a warm embrace may still yearned for (not always) but is unable to cope with the reality of the feelings and uncomfortable sensations it can bring.

In this chapter, I will be speaking of touch in all its varieties, including food, material, toys, people, clothing, animals, footwear and earthly materials such as sand or grass.

I will also touch on (no pun intended!) pressure, this does fall into the proprioception sense too. We have already established that senses overlap and interact and these two are no exception.

Here are a few examples of what can be affected by skin and touch sensitivities:

- hats
- gloves
- jewellery
- Bedding
- Shoes/all footwear
- Tights and stockings
- Socks
- All clothing
- Glasses/spectacles
- Sunglasses
- Scarves
- Suncream
- Shaving/manicures, pedicures/massage
- Night wear
- Touching toys
- Touching food
- Touching humans
- Being touched by humans
- Touching animals
- Creams
- Plaster/band aids
- Nappies/diapers
- Haircuts and hair brushing, tie up etc.
- Tooth brushing
- Dentists/doctors/therapy
- Band aids—plasters, bandages
- Creams/ointments
- Having people or animals close to their bodies/faces
- Blankets
- Hair—long or braided
- Water and baths, showers
- Furniture

- Cooking
- Particular materials

Being sensitive in any of the above areas can be overwhelming especially when you are a tiny baby, young child, non-speaking, and unable to communicate your sensory traumas or process or understand what is happening.

Firstly, I will talk about external touch in their categories and how this can affect an autistic sensitive child's life experience.

As soon as we are born, in most western cultures we are put in clothing from head to toe.

As already discussed, many sensory experiences (although not all) are not realised by others as uncomfortable until the child is developmentally aware of them and or able to express this verbally or physically.

Being a baby means you are unable to tell a parent or carer if an item of clothing, a blanket, carpet, or a touch of a hand is uncomfortable, painful or the opposite of overwhelm—unable to feel it at all unless it is extreme.

Their communication of any discomfort would be limited to screaming, crying, sleeping and shutdown. I have already mentioned that sleep can and is a powerful and valid coping mechanism for sensory overwhelm but because it is a common and natural expectation and part of a young baby's existence, this can be missed as a sensory coping strategy.

Being skin/ touch sensitive means that clothing can be very uncomfortable, children will automatically remove any as soon as they are physically able to if this is where their sensitivity is. If they are unable to because of any physical disability, cognitive understanding, executive functioning issues, maybe dyspraxia or coordination difficulty—you could see behaviours such as crying, screaming, body rashes, hives (large areas of heat and redness) they may squirm, self-harm by means of pinching, scratching, pulling hair, teeth, hairs on their body, headbang, hit themselves and generally be unhappy. They may get very hot, have headaches, feel nauseous, appear hyper active or be lethargic and shutdown possibly wanting to sleep more than usual.

Please remember you will get it wrong for a while, being a detective means you look for clues and try different things out. This is why observing and listening to your children, right from birth is important. Every baby will have different needs as they do not cry for the same reasons. To begin with, it's an elimination process and sometimes a bottle of milk or a distraction will be enough to soothe a young baby until they fall asleep. As they grow into the coming months this tool will decrease in its power and the sensory overwhelm and its awareness can increase. Extreme sensitivity can affect a baby's want to eat or take a bottle, it really does depend on how distressed the baby/child is feeling.

Clothing (including footwear) sensitivity is a powerful and all-encompassing experience. The need to remove such stress and irritant from one's person can be strong which will override the rules and boundaries of nudity in public!

Safety can become an issue too, as in extreme cases if a child is needing to get off their shoes (for example) they could remove them and hurt their feet on concrete or other dangerous footing.

Finding the right materials of clothing for your child is crucial. It can take a while to find the right fabrics, styles, weight, texture and colours. Once you do you will see a huge difference in your child's well-being and behaviours.

Imagine having extremely uncomfortable clothing on all day? Not being able to be or know how to make yourself understood. Crying and screaming doesn't get you the help you need and through no fault of their own, well-meaning parents and carers offer food, milk, toys or cuddles instead?

Think about your own preferences for a moment. What materials do you find uncomfortable? Why are they uncomfortable to you? How do they make you feel? Which part of your body finds certain clothing uncomfortable? Can you wear stripes or patterns, floral, maybe you have colours that you cannot bear to wear, or those that you find comforting?

Personally, I cannot tolerate socks or tights if under a blanket or in bed, it makes my teeth feel itchy and I get very agitated and overwhelmed. I also become hot and claustrophobic. I mostly have to be bare foot and when wearing boots, socks are generally uncomfortable for me. I also find wearing anything tight around my stomach or waist quite uncomfortable, sometimes I can tolerate it but mostly not. Tight clothing is something I struggle with too, I prefer silk, light cotton, soft fabrics and long dresses minimal layers and restrictions. As an adult I can please myself, do what I want and wear what I want. As a child my mother told me I had a nickname "bare bear" I would strip off all my clothes at home regularly. I didn't know this until I was well into my thirties!

Young and non-speaking children cannot tell us verbally if the touch/tactile sense is difficult for them, they rely on us to help figure this stuff out.

Imagine if you are a baby or a toddler who has some of my discomforts and is put into a body romper suit/ baby grow? It might be tempting to put a romper suit, or an all in one on back to front to prevent your child from removing it. If this happened to me, the distress this would cause me is unmeasurable. My behaviour would become heightened in ways of panic and pain. This may sound over the top, but trust me it is a very real and all-encompassing, unpleasant experience, it certainly does not aid sleeping peacefully.

Cutting out the feet (for example) of a romper or baby grow (we call them in Britain) can be all that is needed for a child to feel happier. Or it could be that your child cannot bear to have their bare feet on the ground and wants to wear shoes or socks all the time. Even in the bath or in bed…the feeling of their bare feet on the carpet/floor/grass/sand even water can be very uncomfortable.

Other sensitive skin children prefer to be dressed all the time and having no clothes on, can cause enormous pain and distress. For example: When getting ready for bed or bath time, the removal of clothing into new ones or into a bath can create enough despair for the child to avoid not going to bed or having a bath. The being in bed to sleep may not be the problem, it could be the process prior to being in bed. Changing into other clothing with the air touching their skin can be very distressing for skin sensitive children. Or having hot or warm soapy water with sponges or soaps rubbed onto the skin can be excruciating.

Solutions could be to find a piece of clothing that can be left on like a sun suit in the bath and water shoes. Instead of battling a bath time which can create more fear and problems, find ways that can help ease the stress and intense feelings of skin sensitivity. Remember, each stage is a stepping stone towards a goal.

My son is skin sensitive too—he never wears pyjamas for bed, from a young baby he has not been able to tolerate baby growers he gets extremely hot very quickly too. He preferred to be naked at home and I honoured that as I had similar skin sensitivities, I think it helped me understand the extreme discomforts it can cause. He loved to have soft blankets draped around him when at home or in the garden. As he became older and began developing, I introduced a dressing gown to him. A gown meant he knew he could remove it easily if he needed a short relief, which in turn helped him feel less fearful of wearing one. I had got to know which fabrics he preferred which made it easier for him to cope with. This was around the age of 9, before then he wasn't ready. So, we waited and he carried on wearing his blanket around the house.

It is easy to panic when your child shows no sign of wanting to wear clothes, preferring to strip off. I really do feel the key to helping them cope with clothes on are:

- Allow them to be naked at home if that is what they prefer. Home is their safe space and where anyone can totally be themselves.
- Allow them to have blankets and fabric they do prefer; however unusual you think it is! (Top tip, buy a few spares of any material or type of clothing they prefer)
- Find clothing that is comfortable to them, even if it doesn't "look" trendy or to your liking. (Remember we used Pyjamas for daywear) they were the only types of trousers and tops my son could cope with when he was very young.
- Accept how they like to wear their clothes. (For example, my son likes to pull up his trouser legs to his calves as having them around his ankles is uncomfortable for him) I can now buy him ¾ length trousers and in the winter when he wears boots it doesn't show as much him having the legs pulled up.
- They may not want to wear sunglasses or hats, gloves, scarves, coats.
- They may need to wear the above in all weathers!
- They may need to wear the same clothes everyday (hence buying spares or doubles of everything).
- They may need to wear specific clothes for specific places and experiences.

As already mentioned, an important point to remember is that each stage is a stepping stone. I have found that when things are done in stages and very slowly, it can make all the difference to our children's sensory comfort.

Enabling our children to become comfortable in their own bodies and honouring their sensory needs helps them to feel safe and happier to engage in life. If they are expected to follow social norms or their needs are not read correctly and seen as "bad behaviour", their trust and want to engage with others will remain limited. They may not be able to engage even if they wanted to because their sensory overwhelm is too intense.

I have heard over and over again from autistic individuals how their body and brain often work separately and their sensory overwhelm prevents them from showing understanding of communication or instructions. This can create huge meltdowns and behaviours that are deemed by others as "bad", "naughty", "inappropriate", "dangerous", "unacceptable"; the list goes on and then they end up in a cycle of constantly being misunderstood and their true potential and personality is never seen.

I cannot stress enough to you the importance of honouring your child's sensory needs as much as you can, especially at home. This is why observing and listening to your child's needs and behaviours are crucial in the early years, this early intervention tool teaches you what you need to be able to confidently advocate for your child as they enter nursery and school.

My son, despite his skin sensory needs has always worn clothes at nursery and school and now respite with no problems. He still prefers to wear his dressing gown when he is at home. There are other additional reasons he likes to do this which is related to my earlier point of needing specific clothes for certain places and experiences, the point is, it is his choice. I have no right to tell him he has to do things differently. Especially when I do not know how it feels to him or how uncomfortable it can get.

I truly feel that because I honoured his sensory need to not wear clothes at home or in bed, he could handle wearing clothes elsewhere. I made sure I kept him cool with the materials for his clothing and bedding. It took me a while to figure out that buying Pyjamas for him to wear during the day was the best option. The lightness of the material felt good to him, they were loose and baggy plus I found plenty that had monkeys on them which were his favourite thing at the time. He had (and still does) a more than average natural higher body temperature so he needed to be kept cooler to prevent him from passing out or convulsing.

Now he is older, at respite he wears his clothes all day, not needing to put his dressing gown on other than when he first awakens or after his evening bath. He was given the choice to wear his dressing gown throughout the day if he wanted but he feels comfortable enough to not do so. This part took years to accomplish without pressure or having him feel wrong in any way for his choices.

Now he is an adult the need for him to wear clothes to protect him and his dignity when away from the comforts of home is important. The stepping stone theory is a proven one in all areas of my son's life. Which I will continue to mention throughout the book.

My attitude is, our home space is our sanctuary it is where we all need to be free to be comfortable in every way. He needed that freedom and rest from the sensory overload clothes could cause him and it has paid off massively. I gave him time to get to know himself and what felt nice and what didn't. Enabling him to make choices so that he felt empowered and heard.

Bed times can be tricky for a zillion reasons for our autistic children. My son was no exception when small. One of his main reasons for not being able to sleep was clothing sensitivities. Wearing anything at all when in bed caused him a great deal of discomfort. I weighed up the need to sleep versus my need for him to wear pyjamas, baby growers etc.

This extended to him not being able to not handle wearing a nappy/diaper. This part was tricky because when he was very young and not yet able to use the toilet, he went through a long stage (6 years) of pooping in his room and smearing. BUT despite this, making him wear nappies and romper suits was not an option. It was too uncomfortable for him and his smearing was done for a reason…Eventually, we figured out what that reason was, found a solution and he stopped.

Although not easy, night after night clearing up poo, we ensured he didn't have to wear nightwear back to front or any other kind of method to make him keep a nappy on. He simply didn't sleep and was very anxious, agitated and tired most of the time throughout the day. This broke down our loving relationship and I wasn't prepared for that to continue.

As I previously mentioned, some sensitive children prefer to keep clothes and shoes on at all times. Sometimes coats and hats in all weathers. This can be a comfort for them, or a sensory need, amongst others reasons.

Sensitivities to the Elements

Sensitivities to the different elements is another usual aspect of skin sensitivity. For some children and adults, the sunlight can feel like it is burning into the skin and bones, creating a prickly heat type sensation, which is incredibly painful and uncomfortable. I have experienced it once and my mum allowed me to get drunk it was that bad! I was 15 at the time, so I am not suggesting you give your young children alcohol (more emphasising just how bad it can feel). I have heard that it can feel like a thousand ants crawling over the skin, it is different for each individual.

Sunlight on the skin and face can cause those who suffer to not want to go outside (this doesn't have to be a temperature issue) just sunlight, even winter sun can cause painful sensations on the skin and the eyes. One solution is wearing hats with large peaks and sunglasses. My son cannot tolerate sunglasses but he does love hats, so large peaks on caps is his choice of sun glare solution. Although this isn't perfect, it does help ease the glare. I will continue to offer sunglasses of a variety of weight and styles in case one day he can tolerate them.

Some children will need to have long sleeved shirts/tops and trousers regardless of the temperature outside. Finding the right cool materials can help with this. Baggy or tight clothing can be the issue, or like my son, having his wrists and ankles with gripped clothing is intolerable for him, so he rolls sleeves and trousers up if he has to. He used to also pull his socks down to keep his shins and calves free, now he can wear long socks in the winter to prevent him from getting cold.

Skin sensitivity and what causes my son to have reactions is ongoing. As we come across new textures or creams, materials, plants, foods, soaps, shampoos—anything that will touch his skin in some way we learn pretty quickly what is an intolerance/allergic or sensory response.

Rashes, hives, blotches, redness and dry skin areas are often popping up, some are very temporary, like a food he has touched, for him it is red peppers or certain soap, especially if high in unnatural bleaches or chemicals. We use organic aloe vera soap at home (and now school) as his hands and skin were getting so raw and scratchy, he needed intervention.

Shampoo is another one we have to watch. His hair is super thick, so ensuring his hair is rinsed thoroughly is important if not, his scalp becomes very sore and flaky. It took a while to find the right type of shampoo and knowing how often to wash his hair. We have figured it out—rinse thoroughly, use shampoo twice a week and one that is of a specific brand. So far it is proving successful.

Sore skin is very distracting, even the smallest rash or chaff can feel massive, especially on young skin and on a skin sensitive person. They may also have interoception sensory issues (a chapter coming up) which can enhance physical pain as well as dampen it down.

The same goes for temperature and intensity of water flow and pressure. If the water is slightly hot for my son, his skin comes up red raw as if he has stepped into a steaming hot bath. He has to have the water tepid—he can get very woozy too, which used to lead to seizures. (This was for other reasons) as well as the interoception sensory system. If the water flows too fast, he gets a rash and welts. This information goes into his ICP (Individual Care Plan) and I reiterate the importance of the correct temperature in baths, showers and washing hands.

When he was very young, he did not know he could remove himself from a bath that was too hot for him or uncomfortable—suffering silently until I noticed he was woozy or looking really red on his skin. I emphasise the water wasn't boiling hot, just too hot for him, way too cold for my personal liking—so I learnt to not presume if it felt right for me, it was right for him.

Using your imagination in helping your child meet their sensory needs can be fun. You will almost always find an alternative way or different product/food that will suit your child perfectly. Our children are different, therefore, it's natural that everything will be needed to be done differently in their lives to ensure they thrive in health, happiness and development.

We all know stress and anxiety can be responsible for many illnesses physically, emotionally and mentally. Our autistic children are under an enormous amount of stress every day, for so many reasons. Helping them find ways to reduce it where you can will keep them healthy in body and mind.

I have learnt to always have the bigger picture in my mind, stepping stones that may take anything from moments to years to get to the "bigger picture".

Being patient is a skill my son has taught me which I am grateful for, it has helped me worry less about the future, because I have learnt that it is now that matters, what he needs now, will help him in the future.

Human Touch Sensitivities

Being touched by others can be an uncomfortable experience for many autistic people right into adult hood. This can cause some real emotional distress for a variety of reasons. A big one can be because of the stigma of not wanting to be cuddled or touched by others. (Although sometimes the want is there, but the distress it can cause physically prevents it from being possible)

Being young (a baby) means being held, carried, dressed, fed, bathed, kissed, cuddled and general close proximity to others. On top is talking, eye contact and an expectation to respond.

Imagine being touch and skin sensitive but having to deal with all of that and not having a choice or the words or the understanding to express such discomfort.

When we think in these terms of sensory needs, we can start to realise how much our young children have to deal with. Our understanding of their behaviours and struggles becomes clearer. I know I too would need to scream, kick or run away (for example) if I was constantly overwhelmed by the few sensory difficulties I have mentioned. More so, when we begin to recognise the needs and difficulties our children suffer and remove as many as possible, we see the difference in their happiness and stress levels.

It is worth every moment of waiting, observing, being creative and finding an alternative. The world is big enough for our children's differences—the earlier we can step into this the easier it becomes and the results are undeniable.

Your child may find holding hands difficult, being hugged, hair brushed, washed, put into plaits/braids or pony tails. This could cause pain to them, a panic feeling, a constant overwhelming sensation which enters their bodies inside causing all manner of feelings and discomfort.

Listening and letting go of any of your own needs and expectations is another tool to seeing your child begin to thrive. Remembering the stepping stones of discovery and your child's self-discovery will stand in good stead for changes they may make in the future.

If your child finds giving hugs or being hugged uncomfortable and prefers not to do it, do not take it personally. I too love to be hugged and to give hugs, but my son prefers not to.

He began expressing this once he was able to do so. He was around 12 months when he began wriggling away and squirming from me when we hugged him. However, big firm, pressure, squeezing type hugs with him facing outward were OK. Hugging him from the front/face end was a different experience.

At first, I did take it personally, wondering what I was doing wrong or why didn't he want to receive my love? I soon realised he expressed his love to me and his dad in many other ways. Hugging was simply not one of them and I soon got over it.

Refraining from using shaming sentences even in an unintentional way is a good practise. Remember it maybe that your child would love to be able to snuggle up with you but simply cannot tolerate the intensity or uncomfortableness it brings. Or they may genuinely not care to be hugged, either way they do not need to feel bad for it.

Sometimes a hug can help you feel better emotionally. BUT if you cannot cope with the closeness and intensity of such a cuddle it can make you feel worse on top of then having to deal with the fact you have upset your parents because they want a hug from you.

One solution which worked for my son was to squeeze him. When he became upset for something, usually if he hurt himself or was overwhelmed from another sensory issue, I would ask him if he needed a squeeze. This started as young as 12 months. I would say squeeze in a physical way and use my voice to emphasise the word S Q U E E Z E…initially, I would squeeze his arm until he understood what squeeze meant. I would squeeze him from behind so he didn't get the closeness of my face near his.

This was a breakthrough as he got the comfort, he needed and sensory hit too. (I later learnt about vestibular and interoception sensory systems and why the squeeze felt comforting to him, there will be chapters on both further along in the book.) Plus I got to do the nurturing of taking care of him when he was upset. It wasn't long before he would come up to me and make the "SQUEEZE" sound and make himself go all stiff. This was brilliant as he was communicating to me and requesting the squeeze hugs.

Now at 17, he does receive and give them, although not a favourite thing for him, when I do receive a hug from him of his choice, it is wonderful, he is fully present and I feel his genuine intention. I ask if I can give him a hug and sometimes it's a yes and others it's a no., Of course I accept his choice and freedom to choose.

Another method of hugging is to wrap a blanket around the whole body or make a blanket available so that they can wrap it around themselves and you can hug from behind. I remind you that this is only when your child requests the hug, always their choice and not you insisting on one. (Weighted blankets might be something to consider.)

Choice and acceptance are very important right from the get go. This is not only respectful to them and their body space but also builds trust. Helping your child to say no to things that make them feel uncomfortable is another one of those tools they need throughout life. Non speaking/speaking autistic children can be extremely vulnerable, helping them learn that saying no to being touched in any way can help keep them safe.

We all have inner alarm bells that go off if we feel uncomfortable enough to know we are in danger. If these alarms are ignored or seen as silly, unnecessary or over the top, your child is being taught that their feelings do not matter and worse that their inner voice of sensing danger is incorrect, invalid and not to be trusted.

Resisting their needs and challenges can create mistrust of others and themselves.

Many autistic adults were challenged by most of the examples I have listed, the difference is as adults they have their own choices. Young children by default do not.

Using Hands

This can be a common challenge for skin/touch sensitive children. The nursery is full of textures in play and discovery. Some of which your child may be into massively or seek out sensory soothers to touch which might be seen as inappropriate (like poo) water type solutions if they cannot find actual water (like a toilet bowl) or bottles of detergent and many other "odd" textures and tastes. As long as it isn't unsafe or is toxic, allow them to soothe their sensory needs with such objects and materials.

Sometimes autistic children do not want to touch paint with their fingers or feet, hold a brush or any object for that matter (there could be other reasons for that also)

Nursery and school are filled with creative activities that need the hands to engage with. Your child may need to wear gloves to take part in messy play activities. This could be a solution to a problem which means your child can enjoy painting or sticking etc. with the others. Wearing gloves may not be the solution at all, causing more discomfort. My point is it is OK to do things differently, offer suggestions at your child's school that will help your child however different or unusual that may seem to the staff.

It is also important to point out that your child may enjoy watching others take part in such activities, there is a lot of learning and processing that can happen when watching. My son gets a huge amount of pleasure from watching others engage in a variety of activities. Sometimes he chooses to partake after months of watching, sometimes he chooses to stay away and do something else entirely.

Be mindful that your child gets heard and their needs met and adhered to. If your child does not see joy in painting (for example), then accept that it isn't a joyful experience for them. They may not see themselves as missing out on fun. If it seems they are always on their own doing their own thing, this can mean they are happy with that. Be mindful of the language that is used around your child, no shaming or phrases such as, "you are missing out on all that fun by not taking part" or "it makes me sad that you are not joining in with…" sometimes these kinds of phrases are said to young children as a tool to get them to take part even with good intention. Unfortunately, this can create a deep amount of pressure and shame upon the child.

Alternatives can be to provide a separate tray of sand or water, painting table or other messy play so that your child can enjoy the experience on their terms without the splashing or shrieks of other children's excitement. Some subtle changes in the environment can make all the difference.

Not wanting to be sociable isn't a crime and should definitely not be forced upon. Being in a classroom with others can be socialisation enough for your child, their awareness of what is happening around them is always far greater than you can imagine…the fact they choose to stay away tells you how aware they are.

What can happen (and we want to avoid, moving forward) in nursery and schools is that an autistic child is left in a corner without activities (of their choice) because they cannot take part in what is on offer. Often by offering what they want to do can mean they can enjoy what others are doing from afar whilst enjoying their own activities.

If sensory issues are the reasons your child cannot take part, this is no fault of their own. To deprive them of any activity of their choice whilst the other children are happily enjoying creative arts is unfair and unjust. Equality in school inclusions means offering activities the child does enjoy rather than a one size fits all mindset.

Creams, Plasters, Band Aids, Bandages

There are always times when a young child needs some kind of ointment or plaster/band aid administered from an injury. This is a biggie in our household. My son finds any kind of ointment or plaster/bandage a great difficulty. As soon as I put a cream on or a plaster, he rips it off and wipes it away, or if I am not quick enough, he will eat the Band-Aid before I can get to it.

This has meant wounds take longer to heal and I have gotten very good at finding maximum times when he can have such treatments to assist with wounds. For example, he had a carpet burn on his foot, it was a big one and very sore. I got an appropriate medical kit from the hospital and covered it in the right ointments whenever we went out, as he wore socks and boots. This was the only time he could tolerate wearing a bandage—so he got to have some first aid treatment for a few hours a day. The wound did heal although it took slightly longer than expected.

Although he is very skin sensitive to such things, he also likes me to put some creams on as part of a daily routine! Confusing, right? I believe that this is his way of finding a way for him to get used to having creams on him. This way around, it is his choice and doesn't feel like such an invasion of his body space.

He still rubs it off once I have put it on but he is asking for it to go on his skin, which I see as a positive. Therefore, I go with it. I simply apply the smallest amount, like a pinhead size of a dollop onto his skin. I am hopeful that the bigger picture will be created as he continues to navigate his way through some of his sensory challenges.

Every day is a learning experience for my son within his own sensory needs. As he continues to grow and develop, too have many of his sensory challenges. Some of his needs have completely disappeared whilst new ones have developed.

There is no end point. If your child/adult has sensory processing challenges in any way, the chances are that for the rest of their life they will continue to have them. These may change, become less or more than before; of course, the intensities may increase/decrease—however, they may be with them for life I found the acceptance of these facts made it easier for me to find ways to support my son and you will too.

It takes an imagination and a flexibility to do so, as well as being fun it can help you to find out about yourself and what you do and do not like and more importantly, why. I remind you that all this knowledge you gather about your child is valuable information to pass onto schools, other professionals and family members who may be in your child's life for a long time.

Chapter 10
Visual Sensory Sensitivities

For autistic people, visual sensory processing challenges can affect every aspect of daily life and their experiences for those who have sensitivity in this area. Some are physical symptoms brought on by being visual sensitive, whilst others are physical outcomes because of the visual sensitivity when using the eyes in a variety of settings.

Below is a list that gives *some* of the many examples of how this can manifest for individuals. There will be many more I have not listed here.

- Focus
- Colour identification in shades, actual colour, definition
- brightness
- Distortion of particular patterns and shapes (on floors and carpets) including letters and numbers
- Measuring distance near or far
- Face recognition (face blindness)
- Depth—water, heights so steps, stairs, ladders etc.
- Distracted by visual stimuli (mind scrambled)
- Squints and rubs eyes (more than usual)
- Handwriting is a challenge, such as writing letters the wrong way around, the sizing of letters and the spacing and alignment of letters
- Bumps into things because unable to establish depth and distance

from body

- May find walking in dim lit or dark places difficult,
- May find sunlight or day light difficult
- May find eye contact difficult or impossible.
- May find some colours too bright
- Colour blindness
- Shades and contrasts of colours and imagery
- Distance
- Oscillopsia—when stripes or patterns wobble or move around
- Blindness of some vision in a particular scene or picture
- Blinking at a rapid rate
- Closing eyes for longer periods
- Watery eyes
- Headaches and /or eye aches
- Eye twitches/flickers

This area of sensory processing challenge isn't the same as having an eyesight problem in relation to an optometrist perspective. The eyesight itself can be clear, the tests can show a healthy eye. This is a sensory related state of being.

It is always worth getting an eye test if there are concerns or uncertainties. This can be tricky when a child is very young or autistic and unable to sit still in an optician's chair. Wearing all the special glasses and having lights shone into eyes, being in very close proximity to a stranger, it can feel intense, scary and painful. Therefore, being visually sensitive can mean having any eye test is an incredibly traumatic experience. Add onto other possible aspects of autism, like non-speaking, closeness to others physically, eye contact difficult, being touched and questioned, the list can go on. If you think about the previous chapter and sensitivity to touch and everything that involves an eye test, this can be an impossible reality.

I have been having eye tests since I was 18 months old, so the best part of 50 years and I still find them uncomfortable. I need to prepare myself mentally to "endure" an eye test, especially now with the extra air blasts and beaming lights!

There are other tests you can do at home to collect "data" to take to the opticians (optometrist) so they can assess your child's vision status. Video footage, if possible, could help too. Videoing what tests you are giving your child—distance and size with the toys and activities you are offering them.

Some of the natural testing I have done over the years of my son's life and various development stages are:

Using different coloured items such favourite toys or food (cars, trains, dolls, cups, cloths) for my son it was bath mats that helped me see he could see different colours. He would like them in a particular format, one on top of the other. I put them onto the floor one day and he noticed they were not in the right order for his liking. He moved them around—these bath mats are the same fabric and size the colour is the only difference so I knew he could see different colours. I then went on to try a variety of shades and colours in similar ways to assess his colour recognition skills.

Observing your child with eyesight in mind—do they see tiny specs, bits on the floor? Or only larger objects? Can they see you from a certain distance? Or favourite objects? This can all be done naturally without causing any distress to your child whilst you quietly figure out the basics of their eyesight status. Bearing in mind the list I have given above and the many other sensory reasons your child may not see you at certain distances or depths etc.

Doing these things in a natural way over and over again, using different ways and activities can give you clearer information that you can pass onto the medical professionals. There are times when anyone can have differing eye sight abilities when feeling tired or stressed, poorly or bored to name but a few. Repetition can help build up a useful report of your child's eye health and abilities.

If your child bumps into things or falls over frequently, maybe their eyes water or are bloodshot? These are the type of things you can write down and give to an optician to help them with their assessments. Obviously if your child can cope with a full eye test this will save a lot of work but often an autistic young child finds an eye test particularly difficult to cope with.

My point is to not assume it is because they are autistic that they have poor vision or what looks like poor vision, check it out as best you can to eliminate any health or actual eye problems. Then you know your child has sensory challenges and can focus on that aspect alone.

I have mentioned previously Synaesthesia where senses can become mixed up. Visual stimulations are common in those who have this condition. This is a stand-alone condition that can affect many senses. Visual ones are seeing numbers or letters as colours or seeing sound waves as colours or patterns when certain words are spoken. Some people can have a colour for a day of the week or a number that can have its own sound. I have summed this complex condition up in very few words, which of course tells the tiniest story of the condition. Therefore, I suggest you look up specialist resources on the subject. There are loads of websites that gives detailed and accurate information on all Synaesthesia aspects.

This is where other senses can overlap or affect the visual sensory aspect. I have previously mentioned that if my son has a lot of visual stimulation or a particular set of colours or settings that are not auditory loud, often completely silent, he will still need to close his ear entrances to reduce the sound he hears from the visual stimulation. (This may be a form of synaesthesia) Maybe it is vibration he can hear, or he has such sensitivity he can hear what most humans cannot.

Bear in mind if your child does have visual synaesthesia or a heightened visual stimulus this can become very overwhelming in life as they may see shapes, patterns and colours on top of the sounds they are hearing (often because the aforementioned create their own sounds) This can be distracting making everything they experience more intense or harder to process and understand, let alone respond to.

Concentration could be affected and the ability to focus and hear everything that is being said. Responses maybe slow or non-existent all because their visual sense is so enhanced it takes over everything else.

Do you see how senses can overlap and intertwine? So, what looks like perhaps a hearing issue, could in fact be an overload of visual sensory impact. The ability to hear is perfectly intact but the other sense of visuality is so intense it shuts down the ability to hear in that moment.

Think about your own life, many times when you are in full concentration mode of doing something else and your name is being called quite loudly, yet you cannot hear it. Absorbed deeply into other experiences that are super stimulating shuts out other usually obvious inputs.

I again empathise that observing your child and practising the suggested observational Early Intervention Technique is vital for your child to be understood by you as much as possible through the sensory lens in the early years of their life. This can help you prepare them for any school setting. More so it can help you better prepare teachers on how to support your child so that they have optimal opportunities to thrive at school.

My son's visual sensory awareness is very acute. He sees tiny details and intricacies which can lead to him getting tired by the latter part of the day.

He notices everything, including his peripheral vision. Nothing gets past him. He can spot the tiniest piece of fluff and a single hair on the ground very easily. He can see into far distances too; I know this because I have used various tactics at a variety of distances with him over the years.

When he was younger, he would always look at things from a tilted position, somehow, he saw everything in a slightly different way. He would hold items up to his eyes very close and scan then almost touching his eyelashes. At first, we thought he may have limited eye vision, but we soon realised it wasn't the case. He enjoyed looking at anything he held in minute details. He would also look into my eyes one at a time with his own eye pressed up closely to mine. It was like he had his own magnifying glass mechanism wanting to see things from a distance and then close proximity, detail is very important to him.

Being so visually alert is a great gift but it can create tiredness and overwhelm, which is why down time is important. Decompressing from the day's visual stimulation alone. (Even if they have had loads of fun) being left alone doing their favourite thing, maybe they prefer being in darkness or going on an iPad, watching TV, stimming in any way they choose. (Just some examples) Maybe they like being in the bath for hours? Maybe they want to or need to bounce, climb, lay under a heavy blanket, squeeze things or be squeezed? This part of our children's life is vital to their mental health and wellbeing.

Being hyper sensory alert is extremely exhausting.

Other aspects of visual sensory processing can be to not see the bigger picture or things as a whole. Focusing only on the minute detail, as my son does. This was brought to my attention by an autistic lady I met many years ago. She explained that she went to see a theatre show and absolutely loved the experience. She wanted to watch it again and again. Someone asked her about the plot, she had no idea. Instead, she was focused on the costumes, patterns, texture and colours. She didn't notice the story telling. She was visually stimulated by other things, which meant the intensity of that visual experience was so powerful everything else was dampened down. This was joyful for her, she did not feel she had missed out on anything, instead she got to be visually stimulated and loved every minute of it. For her, that was the part of the show she wanted to focus on. She wasn't interested in the words and singing, the acting or the story.

This could be a reason that an autistic child loves to watch a specific programme over and over again. (There are many other reasons too) but the visual joy of a particular character or setting could be so satisfying and wonderful to your child that they need to watch it over and over. Especially if they do focus on one aspect of the screen for a number of times.

It would make sense then; they would need to re watch many times to get the full picture. Rather than see it as a whole they do so in parts. Repetitive viewing maybe that they enjoy other aspects of the visuality of the scene before them. (It could be for other sensory stimulations such as auditory, remember the senses overlap and work together all at the same time)

Some visual sensory conditions can mean that detail is seen in everything, it is broken down into sections, then the wholeness of something is not noticed. They may focus on one part of an item and "not see" the rest of it. They may start to see more in time, they may not but if we try to hurry the child along or stop their natural process, we risk them losing an important learning and natural enquiry of their experience. Do not be afraid of your child wanting repetition. In fact, relax about it and allow it. This will be for valid reasons, some of which you may never fully understand. Let go of needing to know everything.

Accept their need and want for repetition, (do not worry or see it as a negative to be stopped) rather, knowing for sure that you are enabling their learning experience of self. This is an incredibly important and crucial part of your child's happiness as they grow into adults and engage with other people without you around. A true knowledge of their self and what they need to regulate themselves and thrive in every way. This self-knowledge will help them develop independence and freedom, regardless of the type of care they may need into adult hood.

However, for some autistic people, they can only see the whole picture of an environment. Whatever that environment is, say for example a classroom, they may see EVERYTHING at once, sense it all at once. For now, we are talking about visual stimulation, imagine seeing everything in a room at once? Maybe you cannot, it's a pretty difficult concept to grasp unless you have experienced it. Some folk may deem it impossible to SEE everything at once. Trust me, for some visually sensitive autistic people it is VERY possible and a reality.

That's going to be an overload of sensory input, from the colours, shapes, contrasts, brightness, movement and on and on and on…Now add on auditory, smell, touch? Wow! Suddenly some of the "extreme" behaviours you may have witnessed your child have can be understood more clearly. Trying to cope with that kind of sensory overload and then be expected to engage in ways others expect you to can be an impossible task. Something has to give, an outlet of some kind. Sometimes that outlet will look to others who have no idea what is going on sensorially for the child or autistic adult—a bit over the top or plain weird, unexplainable, for no reason, to get attention, or gain control, have their own way, inappropriate, bad behaviour (I list these types of phrases purposefully, for they are always wrong) There are always reasons—without exception.

Hopefully these chapters of sensory awareness can help you understand why such extreme behaviours happen.

Now, you are beginning to understand how sensory processing in any area can be experienced by an autistic child or adult you can accept why repetition may be needed.

I will talk about this throughout the book, as it can often be misunderstood and seen as a negative behaviour—some forms of therapy or advice is to prevent and avoid an autistic child from repetition, when the exact opposite is deeply needed for many valid and important reasons.

Watching or doing the same thing over and over again is a necessary experience, for visual needs it makes sense to re watch when you are looking at either all detail or only one part at a time, each time you watch or experience something.

Most neurotypical people would not be able to tell you much at all of a particular scene in a movie. What colour was their shirt? What pattern did it have? How many flowers were in that garden? What colour were the cars driving by? They would be focusing a little on the visual but mostly on the story, words, plot, wondering what's happening next.

For many autistic children and adults, they are right in that moment, right there, nothing else is in their minds at all other than that exact moment. That alone is a great gift, focus is relative to one's experience. When anyone says, 'Your child cannot focus or lacks concentration,' I smile, 'if only they knew! I often say to myself!'

What is one person's joy is not another's, this is an important point to remember about your child. They may not engage with experiences in the expected way or how the neurotypical children does. Instead, they are enjoying and engaging in the experiences their way—a way in which they can process the information being shared as optimally as is possible for them at that time. There are many examples of this; not giving eye contact or looking in the direction of the speaking person (teacher) for example.

Maybe your child needs to move around or stay standing up in a classroom setting when everyone else is sitting still? Maybe they need to stim in a way that can look like they are not listening? These are vital traits and needs of your child that you will help them when you learn and accept them.

Passing this factual knowledge on about your child to teachers and other professional bodies who may interact with them into adult hood can help change the old paradigm of autism behavioural understanding, bringing it into the modern neurodiverse acceptance of what autism and sensory processing really means for each individual who is autistic.

Often watching and not engaging for the visually sensitive child/adult is enough. It can bring so much satisfaction and pleasure by watching others take part. Not every activity has to be a hands-on experience for everyone. My son is very visual and auditory so sometimes taking part is simply too much. Watching and listening from a distance is such an intense experience for him it is enough and feels almost as if he is right there doing it.

As I have previously mentioned, these experiences and processing needs can alter and fluctuate as your child grows and develops. Now my son is 17 he takes part in more activities than when he was 10, 6 and 4 years old. BUT he still has many experiences he prefers to stand back from and now I know why. I make sure others understand this so that he can be given the space to watch. If he does want to interact, he will. He has gained plenty of self-learning throughout his life within his sensory systems to feel confident enough to make those decisions for himself.

My role is to ensure that the carers around him know this of him too. I act like an interpreter of his language. Just as if he was speaking French to an English-speaking group of people—they would need an interpreter. As he is a non-speaking communicator and instead a physical, sound and movement communicator, an interpreter is necessary until they are fluent in his language.

There are other conditions like dyslexia that can create visual challenges as well as actual medical conditions. This is an ongoing process, of course as some of the many conditions that affect eyesight and therefore cognitive learning do not become clear until a child reaches particular ages and physical and physiological development stages.

The more you observe your child Interacting naturally with toys, objects, nature, electronics, you will begin to figure out how they see and what their personal levels of needs and therefore support is. There are many choices of sensory visual apps for iPads which are fabulous for children to explore with. By exposing your child to these friendly apps, you will begin to see how your child thinks, problem solves and see's and understands concepts.

Most of my son's apps are sensory based, from words, pictures, science, shapes, puzzles and sorting. Some are about cause and effect like firework patterns and colours creating sounds and shapes. If your child is visually sensitive and / or seeks out highly intense visuals, these apps can be extremely satisfying in many ways. They have all taught me things about my son and his processing systems. Another tip is many of the apps are rated for younger children, do not let that put you off, age-appropriate toys, apps, let it go, if they enjoy it, go with it.

Other tips for using visual aids such as TV, other screens and iPads, apps with visual stimuli are that the sound may need to be lowered or turned down completely. The visual is so "loud" without actual sound. To know what works best for your child, try different volumes. Sometimes visually enhanced children will shy away from activities that are also loud. So, reducing the volume, when possible, may assist them so that they can engage in activities they had previously felt unable to cope with. Checking the brightness levels can make a huge difference to your child's enjoyment of watching TV or looking at iPad/phone screens.

Even if to you the app or activity is better with sound—to your visually sensitive child it can be the opposite. (As is with Auditory sensitivity, they may need it up really loud to soothe the seeking of sound or turned down low to ease the sensory input) So be mindful of this. Sometimes what looks like your child does not want to engage is purely down to needing an aspect of it turned or toned down or up.

Faces can be challenging to see, if out of context. Unless preparation is given. Face blindness is a term often used for this. Some visual recognition is difficult unless there is regular routine meetings and happenings and preparation. The same place and situation can help recognition of that person. Sometimes it is as if the person has only just met you, when in truth they could have met you many times before.

This is (from my research, a common happening for autistic people) seeing people in different settings, or walking down the street can go unrecognised, leaving both parties confused. If someone waves and says hello and the autistic person thinks, *'Who are they? Why are they speaking to me?'* it can appear rude but it is a genuine condition and definitely not meant to be personal.

A familiar face, say of a parent can become unrecognisable if that parent is in a place that was not expected to be seen at.

I have had examples of a child going to a play area with their mum, the dad realised that she had left her keys behind so took them to the location. The child did not expect to see him there and so when he turned up out of the blue the child did not recognise his face. It was only at that moment the parents realised this was a condition their child had. There are situations like this that you may find yourself in and wonder how you could not have known sooner. Some things are difficult to locate until a situation like that arises for you to witness there is an issue.

These are the many reasons why Observational Early Intervention by you is so very important. Your parental/carer's data of your child is the key to their support systems. No one else will know this stuff, you bring this vital information to the meetings, reviews, assessments, diagnosis and development chats, the IEP and EHCP meetings.

Another aspect of this sensitivity can be brightness in general. Bright bold colours can be a sensory seekers joy. However, if you have very sensitive sight, too many bright bold colours can be overwhelming. They can create intense feelings of confusion, nausea, dizziness, headaches, stinging eyes, red eyes, streaming eyes, continuous blinking or complete shutting of the eyes. Such overwhelm can feel like your head will explode—sounds may develop that are loud and uncomfortable. Your child may hold their hands over their faces, run away, hide, cover themselves up with clothing, shout, shrill, try and break whatever is causing them discomfort or pain, cry, lay down, run away or try—these are just a few examples of how intense the discomfort equals the efforts taken to rid themselves of that pain.

Having bright lights on at home can create the aforementioned behaviours because it is too bright, almost like having a torch shone directly into your face. This can be the same for lighting in schools, halls, nurseries, hospitals, doctors, dentists, as well as the TV being too bright, the fluorescent lights in particular can be excruciatingly bright as well as loud!

Sunlight can be another intense sensory experience for visually sensitive children and adults. Creating physical experiences such as prickly heat, burning, itching, tickling, a feeling of swelling up and unable to regulate breathing, feeling like they will suffocate in the sunlight or heat. Tiredness and drowsiness (sometimes passing out) can happen instantly when exposed to heat or sunshine.

For the visual sensitive (and skin sensitive), sunlight can be the reason to not want to be outside in nature. If you cannot see through the brightness of the sunshine, you cannot enjoy any activity or experience outside. My son finds sunlight tricky. He cannot bear to wear sunglasses but he will wear a hat or long peaked cap. This helps reduce the amount of sunlight into his eyes. He prefers to have his skin covered up—unless he is in the water or is highly stimulated with other joyful activities. He needs to wear long-sleeved shirts even in the highest temperatures of summer. So, he wears a light cotton shirt over a t-shirt just like a jacket or cardigan. This prevents him from overheating and passing out (his internal body system is particularly sensitive to heat), as previously mentioned, he has interoception sensory difficulties.

When an autistic child is either young, non-speaking or cannot figure out what is bothering them because it is too overwhelming, it is up to you to figure this stuff, then find ways to reduce or enhance the environment to give your child relief. Which means perhaps experimenting with different wattage and brightness of lights until you find the right balance. Creating the perfect environment for your child's sensory needs makes a huge difference in their happiness, health and mental well-being especially when at home.

This can be the case for visually seeking people, needing bright, dazzling, sparkling, flashing, particular-coloured lights.

It all takes time; please remember you are not going to figure all this out overnight. It can take years to finely tune all the sensory needs of your child, so bit by bit, day by day and you will learn the language of your child's sensory makeup.

All behaviour is communication therefore when your senses are so finely tuned that a simple light bulb can create a sensation of giddiness, nausea, headaches or even a feeling of blindness (just some possible examples) your behaviour can understandably become stressed and manic. It could seem to the outsider to be unreasonable, trust me if behaviours are loud, extreme and frantic then that is how your child is feeling. Always listen and take it seriously. You may take a while to figure it out but when you do and you see a difference in their demeanour and their happiness—patterns will emerge then you will be on the road to understanding your child senses the environments are in and how their personal sensory systems work.

On the other end of heightened sensitivity is under sensitivity where pastel colours, certain tones, shapes or patterns can be difficult to see or separate. Walking around in dark places or low-lit rooms, with lamps may be difficult. Maybe they cannot see certain objects, toys and blankets that are right in front of them. They may find walking up or down stairs very difficult or walking on escalators (this is one of mine) shapes and images may move around, some look like they are 3rd and 4th dimensional which can create falling over or bumping into things. (There are other reasons this could be happening like interoception and vestibular sensory challenges) which are separate chapters.

They may simply stand still and not want to move in darkness or low-lit places as suddenly they cannot feel or see themselves within the space (this can also be vestibular sensory issue) visually they may not see objects in a lower lit environment, depth and distance can become unclear causing them to bump into furniture and fall down curbs and steps.

Sometimes looking at something for long periods of time can create a fragmented view of things. A bit like a dyslexic person who sees letters or patterns jumping around a page or board…looking at faces or TV or screens can become distorted or the images can move around where you cannot make sense anymore of what you are looking at. This can be another reason why wanting to rewatch certain TV shows or apps can happen, or not wanting to watch TV or engage in board work or reading, drawing or any close-up creative activities.

Eye contact is a huge topic of conversation around autism. Luckily for the neurotypical person, whether parent or professional there is an incredible amount of information on this subject that has been devised by actual autistic people. My advice is to source this information. Specifically, from the autistic humans of this world. Eye contact and whether it can be tolerated is a person-by-person reality.

Like other sensory needs and challenges, it can fluctuate and change depending on many things. One of these factors can be the familiarity to another person. Sometimes knowing someone well can make it is easier for an autistic person to give some eye contact, after all nobody gives 100% eye contact, we all look away from and around a person's face when having a conversation. Otherwise, it becomes staring.

Eye contact can be a painful experience, literally physically painful. Creating headaches, dizziness, nausea, dry throat and heart palpitations to name just a few. It can feel extremely scary and claustrophobic having to look at someone close and intensely, as well as having another person look intensely into their eyes, all of this can create deep feelings of discomfort.

If visually sensitive, looking into someone's eyes whilst they are speaking can be impossible. This can cause a person to not hear or understand what is being spoken. The visual stimulation of the face added to the sound and tones, words and demands of a voice can all break down into an impossible incoherent mess. Looking away, even closing eyes can help the autistic person hear and understand what is being spoken.

This knowledge is becoming more widespread and more importantly accepted by non-autistic professionals and therefore is no longer seen as something that needs to be fixed or challenged. However, there are still remnants of those who feel working on eye contact is necessary. Some organisations will suggest you work on eye contact skills and strategies with your child if they find it difficult.

On my son's original Statement of need, one of the actions was to have a staff member hold his face towards the person who was speaking to him! Back then I was not emotionally strong and did not pay enough attention to the details of what was written in such documents. I naturally assumed that the care and practices offered to my son would be suitable for him. NEVER is touching a child's face and keeping them locked there OK, there is no valid reason as to why this is a good or beneficial aspect to a person's life. It creates anxiety, stress for all the aforementioned reasons as well as many others that are unique to that person. Understanding a person can hear and process clearly without giving eye contact is necessary for a positive relationship to be created between the autistic person and therapist/teacher etc.

From the countless numbers of autistic people who experience eye contact as challenging in some form or another, I would say there is enough evidence to eradicate the belief that eye contact is necessary to learning and listening. It simply is not a truth, instead a neurotypical view and need to have the person they are speaking with, look at them. Especially in an educational setting or 1-1 therapy session.

This is an outdated and nonsensical expectation therefore, as an advocate for your child/adult, you can instead educate on why eye contact is an unimportant aspect of the session. Ensure this is accepted and acknowledged by the adults and professionals around your child/adult so they are not subjected to any exercises that insist on them giving eye contact during any interactions. If you need further evidence and reasons why eye contact is difficult as well as unimportant when it comes to listening or absorbing information have a look on some of the social media groups led by autistic people. There are many documents and personal stories on such topics.

Some autistic adults have learnt to look at foreheads or eyebrows or just above the headline. But this can still be uncomfortable for some and causes anxiety when socialising or communicating with other people. This then creates a deeper anxiety and can prevent a person to want to meet with others in any capacity in case they are expected to give eye contact. This can be a reality for your child going to school or nursery. Being constantly told to give eye contact purely because the other person needs you to isn't a good enough reason to insist on it happening.

Let it be a choice thing, trust that your child is getting what they need or more importantly what they can process at that particular time/stage in their lives. Your insistence of others refraining from expecting eye contact of your child will help non autistic people accept that not being looked at when speaking does not mean they are not being heard or listened to. In fact, it means the opposite.

Like other sensory needs this will fluctuate and change depending on a person's individual needs. Tiredness can have an effect on whether eye contact can be given. What is going on around them, like other noises and activities can mean eye contact is impossible.

Think about a time for yourself when you have had to close your eyes or look away from someone to concentrate on what is being said to you. Often it happens to neurotypical people when there is too much going on or a particularly difficult question is being asked. Closing eyes or looking away somehow helps one concentrate and find clarity in thought.

Of course, there are autistic people who can give eye contact without any issues or discomforts, for others it is an infrequent challenge—depending on the reasons already mentioned.

For those whom it is, please accept it and let go of the need to please others. You may well be surprised by how much your child can see, hear and process without looking at another person's face compared to when they are made to give eye contact.

Visual sensitivity either enhanced or underwhelmed is, as you have learnt—a major aspect in daily life. It can be the blockage to engaging in its many experiences for your child/adult.

I hope that this glimpse into the visual sense and how processing with sensitivities in this area can be has given you a good foundation of understanding.

Chapter 11
Interoception Sensory System

The interoception sense is one that I hadn't heard of it until I became interested in our sensory systems, seems crazy really when it is an integral part of our bodily function and well-being. Back when I initially began studying the senses in a meaningful way, this one was not spoken about within the autism diagnosis processes. More recently, it is now known amongst some agencies that can be involved in an assessment process for anyone seeking a diagnosis of either sensory processing disorder or autism.

For those of us who have a balanced sensory system and a neurotypical brain, this sense flows along without having any thought needed on how it works, or that it exists at all.

In this chapter, I will give a brief description of its functions but urge you to further research it on more specialised websites and resources if any of this rings true for your child or client. I will be talking about how this sense can affect autistic children and adults who have challenges with it from a practical perspective.

The interoception sensory system is, in broad terms, a sense that constantly tells our bodies how it feels. This can be subconsciously or consciously, it never stops asking and checking, it is a very busy and important aspect of our sensory system and well-being.

This includes functions such as:

- Toileting needs (full/empty bladder, bowels)
- Food needs (hungry, thirsty, full up, quenched)
- Pain Hyper or hypo
- Internal body discomfort/pain and functioning—including all organs
- Temperature both inside and outside of the body
- Self-regulation challenges
- The autonomic nervous system activity related to emotions—regulation and expression

This looks like a short list in comparison to some of the others in previous chapters yet when we look at its contents—it becomes clear how huge this sense is. If affected, it can create enormous challenges for the child/adult, some of which can be harmful to their health, personal safety as well as their mental and emotional well-being.

Toileting

On average, a neurotypical child will begin the early stages of toileting around 2–3 years old. There are many strategies suggested in childcare books, depending on the child and their environment which may govern their success.

This also depends on how long the carer/parent is willing to wait until the child feels at ease and comfortable enough to become fully diaper/nappy free and to be able to monitor their own toileting needs completely independently.

It is a huge stage in a child's development, a great deal of attention is e created around this and how this process is handled will affect their emotions and self-esteem. Whilst a large majority of toddlers cope quite well with the demanding and intense process of toileting practises, many do not.

Many parent/carers are innocent to the negative impact intense toileting practises can have on a child if they are not ready emotionally, physically, mentally and developmentally. Sometimes too much focus can create anxiety around toileting making it more difficult for the child to naturally "go" some develop a fear of disappointing a parent if they cannot perform on demand or if they have accidents during this transition period.

Often once the process is started there is a need from the carer to get it right as quickly as possible. This may be due to pressures from Nursery and preschool regulations. Many schools and nurseries prefer a toddler to be toilet independent as soon as possible. So, if they are not by the time, they are 3 years old, pressure builds as school start dates loom, this adds pressure to the parent/carer, which can flow onto the child through no conscious fault of theirs.

There are tick charts, sticker books, reward charts, negotiations such as "if you do…you can have…" treats and promises made and given, singing potties, musical potties, flashing toilets, clapping of hands and the parents/carers telling anyone who will listen what their child has achieved in toileting that day in order to encourage the child to get to grips with independent toileting.

Language changes towards the child and suddenly they are "big girls or boys" and are wearing big girl or boy knickers/pants/ underwear. Suddenly the word baby becomes a negative, 'You are not a baby, are you? Well then you can use the toilet/potty as only babies have nappies/diapers.' All of this is done with good intent but sometimes carers can get carried away and forget there is a child with emotional needs too.

Of course, I am exaggerating slightly but hopefully you get the point I am making of the intensity the toileting teaching experience can be.

Whilst most of it has a positive effect and the child quickly learns how to tell when they need the toilet, meaning nappies and diapers are a thing of the past, it isn't necessarily the case for all children, particularly autistic children.

If your child has interoception sensory difficulties, none of the mentioned methods will work, instead the child may shut down, become withdrawn, angry, lash out, hide, increase their toileting in secret, unconventional places or they may withhold their pee or poo. This can cause physical health and emotional problems.

Interoception sensory related toileting issues can be difficult to pin point if the carer isn't aware what this sense is. It isn't something we learn about unless our careers or personal health warrant knowing about it.

Usually a psychologist, psychiatrist, nurse, doctor and an Occupational therapist will have some knowledge of this body function. Often it can take a while before a parent or carer feels it necessary to seek professional help, meanwhile the child could be internalising and suffering emotionally depending on how long the toilet training regime has been going on for.

Interoception senses tells us when we need to use the toilet. That feeling we get when we know we need a wee, even at the very first stages, it informs us a wee is brewing so we can start looking for a place to pee! This message doesn't get through to a child or adult with difficulties in this area, therefore disabling them from knowing when they need to go.

It just cannot happen, which means a child will go wherever it can, whenever the body can no longer hold onto it. This will be as big a surprise to the child as it is to anyone else, not knowing you need a wee until you are actually doing it, is a strange experience and if not handled with compassion it can cause shaming issues and anxiety.

When toilet practises are put in place that a child cannot meet, despite the thrills and praises, gifts and star charts available to them this can be frustrating for the adult and soul destroying for the child and very confusing.

More than likely a young child will not know why they cannot grasp the concepts that are expected of them by their parents or carers. The body and brain are not communicating in time to get to a toilet or a potty. They only know they need to pee or poo when it is actually happening, or at the very last minute, so no heads up, no internal feeling that says, 'Oh, I need the toilet.' Certainly not enough time to get to a potty or toile, resulting in accidents happening in all manner of public places.

This is an issue that can stay into adult hood, resulting in the need to wear incontinence knickers or padding to maintain privacy and dignity when out and about in public.

What can look like a behavioural or intellectual issue is in fact an internal sensory system malfunction. Part of that system isn't working, the sound button if you like is turned right down. If you cannot feel when you need to go, how can you avoid wetting or soiling yourself? It is impossible.

Whilst many autistic children can toilet independently there are many who cannot either ever or when the milestone child development charts is typical of a child of a certain age.

This is definitely worth investigating as a possibility if you find your child or client has issues in toileting. There are many other reasons why an autistic child may not be grasping the independent toilet skill but interoception is certainly a high factor. The sooner you know if this is the issue, the less stressful toileting practises can be.

It may mean that you put off toilet independence for a few more years and wait for their individual development in this area to grow. Usually this is the case by ages 7–10, where autistic children with this sensory difficulty have managed to become completely toilet independent or partially so with the aid of incontinence support clothing.

Occupational therapists are usually the support required for this area as they can help the child learn about their internal system and help you support them. There are also the groups led by autistic communities who are happy to offer advice and support with this particular situation.

Finding ideas that can positively support your child's sensory needs can make a difficult process that bit easier. The very nature of toileting can be a messy experience if accidents happen, as well as keeping your child's dignity intact if in public places as well as in schools and colleges.

Like the other senses, as well as being hyposensitive they can also be hypersensitive, which means in this scenario that your child may feel they need to poo or pee a lot. This could be because their hyper alert interoception sense is super tuned to that aspect of its bodily function. They might only poo a tiny bit or do a very small wee (this is just an example) and again as a reminder there are many other reasons a child may feel the need to go to the toilet often.

It is advisable to get them physically checked to ensure that their health is intact, particularly infections in the bowels or bladder. Once you know that aspect of them is fine, you can then be sure of the sensory interoception being the reason for such difficulties and sensitivities.

If an OT (occupational therapist) carries out an official assessment that can diagnose sensory processing difficulties, it can go into the child's EHCP, ILP, IEP, SON (statement of needs) so the school has to adhere to the care plan and support your child during the school day in the ways that are outlined in their statements.

I could write a whole book on toileting and autistic children to be honest. For now, though I am talking about toileting issues around this particular sense.

Food and drink—hunger and thirst—empty and full

Eating issues are not uncommon in autistic children, or any child actually. Most have challenges with food and taste, texture, colour, smell, shape and quantities during their lives. This is another tricky area where it can be difficult to identify that the child has interoception issues around eating and drinking.

For some, this means they do not feel hungry—it simply does not happen and so eating is a strange concept. I am sure you yourself have at times not felt hungry for some reason or another and no matter how much you want to eat a particular meal you cannot bring yourself to do it. If you did force yourself, you might end up gagging, vomiting or the very least feel nauseous at the thought of eating something you might ordinarily enjoy.

Imagine if this was the case for you all of the time? Worst still, not knowing why? If this isn't understood by the carers and adults in the child's life, they may be seen as being "picky or stubborn" eaters (a phrase that is used often to describe difficulties in eating) you may think they have a stomach issue or digestive problem.

Like the toileting issues it can be a long and arduous road to finding out exactly why your child isn't wanting to eat or show any interest in food whatsoever. Yet everybody needs to eat, so eventually the child will because they start to feel the need to survive as their bodies shut down. Only when extreme feelings of hunger kick in can a hyposensitive child recognise the need to eat. Please be aware that this may not happen naturally for the child, starvation and dehydration can occur if the adults around them do not monitor their food and drink intake.

These big problems can occur when a child is very young and has this sensory impairment. Hunger or thirst may be felt, eventually at a crisis point and with the lack of nutrition and energy of food, they may get to passing out, feel giddy or very tired, lethargic and disorientated. They may feel very anxious and hyper active. Their emotional state may be fraught, they may start screaming, crying, stimming intensely towards themselves particularly, they may sense something is wrong but cannot tell or express what it is.

The opposite to not knowing when they are hungry can happen with this sense where they do not feel full up. That bloated feeling we get when we have had enough to eat, that satisfying feeling of knowing you have fuelled up enough and can stop eating. For some children and adults, this is the part that is missing, the message of OK, we are full now, replete, no more food is required, is the message that is missing or is very low and quiet.

This can look like the child is being greedy, constantly asking for food, perhaps taking others food, and not taking no for an answer, they may cry or become angry. They may begin to hoard food and hide it so they can continue to eat in the fear that someone will take the food away and tell them they have had enough when they simply cannot feel full. There are of course other reasons why an autistic child may want to continue to eat and eat, they may be for medical reasons or other sensory reasons. The taste/mouth sense can certainly have an effect on how much foodstuff is needed to satisfy the need to feel things in the mouth as well as the proprioception sense, needing to feel pressure or sensations in the mouth/teeth/jaw areas, (more of that in later chapters.) this sense is definitely one that can affect a child's ability to recognise when they are completely full up.

The concerns and possible problems of not being able to feel full up are:

Possible constipation or excessive loose stools, stomach cramps, indigestion, headaches, thirst, obesity, extreme lethargy, hyperactive (depending on what they are eating) developing food intolerance and allergies and vomiting are a few examples.

Being thirsty and knowing when to drink and when to stop is also affected which can have serious health issues if left undetected. Dehydration can be an issue worse still long term, this can have serious health complications. Short term, feeling dehydrated can make someone feel rather unwell.

If you have been dehydrated, you will know what I speak of, if you have not here is a short list of potential symptoms of dehydration from minor to severe.

Headache, dizziness, tired, poor vision, faint, back ache (kidney pain) unable to urinate or very strong urine, urine infections, disorientation, unable to focus or concentrate, tearful and angry. If this goes on for a while, developing long-term dehydration can be critical. Whilst we can get some liquid from our food if your child has interoception sensory difficulties that affect both food and drink this can be especially difficult and dangerous.

Equally excessive drinking can create some issues too, especially if not enough salt or sodium type foods are consumed, a lack of salt because of over dilution in the body can create faintness, low blood sugar, giddiness, hyperactive behaviours, bladder control issues or kidney pain.

If you suspect your child may be experiencing challenges in this particular area, until you can attain an assessment by an Occupational Therapist or other health professional you could offer your child intermittent drinks. Make it fun, be creative, remember if they do not feel the need to drink, they will find the concept difficult to grasp. So, buying their favourite characters cup or use a fun straw if they can manage the sucking function. Give them ice-lollies you make at home with flavoured water. You can use real fruit juice in ice-lollies which are great fun for kiddies, if they can handle the flavour.

My son has issues with drinking and eating—even now I have to prompt him to drink water. We make it fun and he loves/prefers to use a straw. He simply wouldn't drink enough fluid in a day to be healthy if he wasn't given prompts to drink, we also include it as a routine, scheduled water drinks to ensure he gets a good minimum at the very least. This has resulted in him having a big beaker/glass of water into his daily routine which over the years he has been able to grasp. This means he gets 4–5 pints of water a day. He is 17, so needs more fluid and he doesn't like any other type of drink.

You can create water-drinking opportunities in play too, as long as the water is clean and has no colouring in it that may cause problems, using water play in various ways can mean your child gets some fluid inside them. Sticking with water or very diluted juices can help with maximum hydration without the other chemicals or additives which can make it easier for the body to utilise the fluid for organ health. Sometimes the additives in some drinks can create dehydration which is what you would be trying to avoid.

For excessive drinking, you can help manage their intake by using similar beakers and cups of their favourite characters creating games so that they do not feel punished or bad for needing to keep drinking. Over time if managed carefully there is every chance that they will learn how to self-regulate safely, when they are educated about their bodies and its many differing needs. If this is difficult—making drinks and meals as part of their routine (using a social board) can help keep an eye on how much they are drinking and eating.

It is important to seek medical advice regarding organ health as well as perhaps a dietician who will have more skills and ideas on what fluids, mineral and vitamins your child may need.

Feeling Pain

This sense can create issues around pain in and outside of the body. Like with the others this can be tricky to recognise until things start getting out of hand, sometimes it takes an accident or incident to realise this is an issue.

For some children and adults, this area of the interoception sensory system can mean they do not feel pain until it is at its most extreme, or certainly not until it becomes dangerously painful or harmful. There are varying degrees in how much pain each human feels as pain thresholds vary from person to person too. This though is more about simply not feeling pain rather than tolerating it for periods of time.

Some of us for example, can hold a hot plate, whilst another may need to use a tea towel. I know people that can drink hot tea whilst others (including myself) have to wait a while for it to cool off before drinking it.

For interoception issues around pain, this can be extremely dangerous. We all manage our physical safety by feeling temperatures or weight (for example). We instinctively know when something is becoming too hot because we feel it, we pull away. For an interoception hyposensitive person pain will be difficult to feel. Whilst a hypersensitive person will find the slightest touch or warmth more painful than the average person.

My son has hypersensitivity with heat, especially when in the bath or any water. He heats up incredibly quickly from the inside out and becomes faint and floppy. In fact, this was one of his triggers for seizures. Now he is older he has become self-aware of this, because he has had plenty of managed experiences in the bath with varying temperatures so he has slowly learnt to self-manage. He can still only tolerate tepid bath water; I find it too cold but it is perfect for him.

The difference now is he can tell me by lifting himself out of the water slightly that the water is still too hot for him rather than staying in the bath and suffering, as he did when he as younger. He looks at me and waits until I acknowledge what he is telling me. We are currently working on helping him to turn taps on and off himself so he can become more independent and safer when bathing.

When he was younger, I had no idea this was an issue for him. He was always in water, whether the bath, rivers, water play in the garden or the sea. He began getting floppy and faint when he was in the bath—I had no idea why because to me the water was not hot to touch and his skin was not red, which would have helped me see the water was too hot for him. It took me a while to realise it was the temperature in the bath. He is also sensitive to heat with the sun and stuffy rooms.

So, it is important to listen to a child or adult who says they feel the temperature is too hot or cold (whatever the case may be) even if to you it isn't they will need to be heard so that they can continue to self-regulate their desired temperatures.

There are bath thermometers on the market that can be put onto the bath so a visual can tell you when the water is at the desired temperature. You can also have special temperature control put onto taps to ensure the hot water tap stays at a safe and required heat, perfect for your child.

This may include issues with the temperatures of food and drinks. If the food is hot in actual heat, they may find it painful to eat if they are hyper sensitive to heat, if they hypo, they may not feel that a food or drink is scorching hot and can end up burning their mouths or gullets when swallowing food and drink. It can also be the reason why a child may not want to eat at all if they are unable to express the burning sensations they have when eating and drinking, they may have no other way of communicating that other than to stop eating altogether, however hungry or thirsty they may be.

Remember what is hot or cold to you will not be the case for your sensitive child. Most of my son's food is eaten tepid or cold. He will busy himself with routines whilst his food cools down. Personally, some of the food he needs to be cooler I would not enjoy. But it is not up to me to decide whether he should eat his food hot or not.

My role is to ensure his food is safe to avoid food poisoning and that's it. I would rather he ate his food happily and stress free than concern myself with whether I think his food is the "right" temperature.

The other end of pain thresholds is the inability to feel pain until it is at an excruciating (to you) level or more importantly a dangerous level, which can be very harmful. For example; if a bone is broken, or a head is whacked on a wall or floor, they cut themselves or lean onto something sharp or hot, maybe scrape their skin or burn themselves on carpets or slides. If clothing is too tight or hair bands are tied up tight and cause headaches and tension. Maybe their shoes are tight and rub, causing blisters, sunburn can be an issue if they do not feel the burning of their skin, they could become very poorly indeed. Bites and stings may not be felt or biting their own tongue, pulling off finger nails by biting too low down.

My son has difficulties in this area, he processes pain very differently to the typical person. When he was young, he would laugh when he was in pain (this took a while for me to figure out) I am very glad I did as it has saved him from having some serious situations regarding hurting himself further. Lately though he is experimenting with pain and how deep it can go for him.

Throughout the book I have talked about how an autistic child continues to develop and grow and a part of that is discovering their ongoing sensory processes, for they also fluctuate and change throughout age and puberty stages.

My son is now a young adult and he has begun to investigate how to feel out pain and his threshold within it. This has resulted in him pulling out his toenails! It started slowly, bit by bit—until he pulled off a whole toenail. This was very painful, as he processed this intense pain, I could see he was learning about his limits as well as feeling what pain was.

He is also very routine based in all areas of his life. Pulling out toenails was no exception, he creates routines very quickly and this became a part of his nighttime routine, during a particular activity. This is something we are still working on together—to help him stop as he had pulled out six of his toes nails out which has resulted in a lot of lint, bandages and antiseptic potions. As he finds plasters and bandages difficult to cope with, this has been a challenging time. I am hopeful that he has learnt for himself within his body the deepness of pain that he has never been able to feel before, experiences will help him know to stop doing it! So far this seems to be the case and he has stopped this behaviour.

I have heard stories of people who have had numerous broken bones and fractures in their feet, hands, arm and legs yet no one knew because they did not register the pain, no hobbling or complaining, so it got missed until someone noticed something and an x-ray revealed the truth.

If a child with this sensory issue has tummy pain or a headache, toothache, any kind of internal pain or discomfort, some of those pains could become critical to their health, so it's really important to know about this sensory issue to help monitor your child more closely and more importantly as they grow and develop help them to self-regulate and become more safety aware.

For example, your child may not feel an earache or toothache or may feel something in a very minor way, yet in fact the earache is at infectious stage and is showing other signs such as giddiness or lethargy. Their mouth may become swollen before you know they have an abscess on their gum or tooth.

The flip side is of course hyper sensitivity to pain (this can be an issue for me) so what might look like a gentle knock to the leg or a slightly warm plate (for example) can feel incredibly painful to a hyper sensitive interoception sensory system. If a child is screaming in agony when all that seemed to have happened was a soft bang on the head or a tiny graze, this can be experienced as excruciatingly painful and needs to be treated as such. Telling a child that it isn't THAT bad or that it doesn't hurt THAT much can be traumatic and confusing to the child experiencing the feeling they are having. The dangers of being told that you are not feeling something you clearly are by the adults in your life can result in not being self-aware of dangers and not trusting your own feelings and judgements.

It is always tricky to know when a young child—whatever their neurotype is if they are in pain internally. For example, if they have organ discomfort or more serious disharmonies going on in their bodies. Added to this challenge is if your child is unable to feel the pain that can alert us as carers to getting the right treatments as quickly as possible. One that springs to mind is appendix—this can be extremely painful and if burst can be critical. If pain is not processed until it is at its maximum, things can get scary.

This chapter can seem a little overwhelming and worrying, if there is awareness of this sense and being able to catch on as early as possible if your child has this particular sensory issue, you will naturally get used to being super alert to your child's physicality and wellbeing.

As the child ages and becomes more frequently out of your care, whether that is when they are at school or in a residential college or home. It is better for them to have some independence in their knowledge of what feels safe, pain free and pleasant for them in all areas of their lives, from eating to bathing to exploring and engaging with activities, particularly when engaging with others. This will enable their autonomy in choices that are best for them. This area of their sensory needs is vital knowledge when they are away from home, until they are at the stage where they can manage this successfully and safely on their own—other carers and teachers will need to know about any interoception needs—especially when they stay all day or overnight.

Like with all the senses, part of this books intention is that by you learning, understanding and accepting your child's sensory systems, you can, in turn help them learn about themselves. This can help them be freer in their lives. Some of you will have children that will always need some form of living support into adult hood (as will my son), whilst others will become semi or completely independent but will still have some intense sensory needs.

By helping them learn what is both safe and comfortable to them in all areas of their lives, you will ensure they can live as pain/stress free as possible. More so, you can help them recognise when something is not right for them and they need to remove themselves from an environment, experience or person before they go into a shutdown scenario or are hurt.

Some of what I have written in this chapter will cross over to the sense of touch and pain, some touch related experiences can feel intensely painful if for example the blanket is too heavy it may genuinely hurt them. If the material in their t-shirt is irritating, it can be a feeling of intense burning or itching. For the outsider looking in, this may look like an extreme (even unnecessarily so) reaction to an uncomfortable feeling. Yet to the sensory sensitivity of your child the pain is real and needs to be accepted and honoured.

Feelings/emotions and expressing them—feeling fearful—a sense of danger.

The internal message, we receive—when our bodies tell us we are in danger may be affected if this sense is compromised in any way. It may create a feeling of ongoing heightened panic or unease as well as a dampened down ability to know when we are in any danger.

The ability to feel when something isn't right for us, or is causing distress in one way or the other is crucial to our self-safety monitoring. It is how we know when to say no to something or someone, or to ask them to stop doing something we do not like because it physically hurts or emotionally does not feel good to us. This area of the sensory system being affected can enhance the person's personal safety. It can leave them open to experiences that could be internally and externally uncomfortable, painful or harmful but are unable to express this clearly enough for the outsider to recognise.

It is advisable that any therapy sessions a person has is given when parent/carers are also present. Certainly, in the first few weeks/months so that the therapist can be guided by them (it is they who will have the knowledge of what behaviours are being communicated at any moment during a session, especially those of discomfort, stress as well as happiness and joy)

If you are unable to be in the room (there isn't really a valid reason why this should be the case, unless the child/adult themselves expresses this), you should be able to see through glass what is happening and or at the very least have a sound monitor to hear what is being said. (Although I suggest being visually or physically present is better.) This enables you and the therapist/professional to work together to ensure you are all supporting the child in the best way that honours their needs and requests.

This sense can affect a person's regulation and expression of emotions. If they are unable to feel their internal organ pain, any outside body pains (including being touched) as well as hit or bumped by something or by being touched by another person or clothing (for example) they will not be able to express emotions that one would usually be able to do.

If hyposensitive they may not cry, scream or express an emotional response to help a carer know they are hurting. If hyper sensitive, they may express their pain by screaming loudly which may cause the carer to think perhaps a bone has been broken (for example) when in fact they are physically OK but still feel pain in adherence to a broken bone level of pain.

Either of these can be dangerous for the child, especially if a bone is broken (for example) and the child cannot express that level of pain because they simply cannot feel it on that level.

Some children get muddled about their feelings and so expressing how they feel may be confusing for both the child and the carer.

For example, my son would often laugh if he was hurt, when he was around 4 years old, another child was jumping on his back during a soft play adventure. They were only about 5 years old too, he was merrily jumping on my sons back as he lay face down on the ground, whilst this was happening my son was laughing very loudly. Of course, the other child, being only 5 thought he was enjoying the experience and continued to jump because my son's behaviour said, 'This is fun!'

It was only because I recognised the type of laugh my son was expressing—it was slightly different to his genuine happy laugh, however to a stranger's ear it sounded like a regular laugh. I knew he was in trouble even though I couldn't actually see him as I was not in his eye line. I ran and quickly stopped the boy from jumping on his back. My son was a little traumatised by the whole event but had got muddled about how it felt and how to express it.

I learnt that my son would often laugh when hurt or when he was sad by just observing his behaviours very closely, right from when he was a baby. I have previously mentioned, I am a trained nursery nurse and a huge part of our training back then was observation of children in various play activities, developmental and age stages in a vast variety of situations and scenarios. It really is an excellent learning tool; you learn so much from observing and listening—without actually engaging.

If my son had been with someone who did not know this "laughing" sound was in fact his pain sound, he could have been seriously hurt. These are the golden bits of information you can learn about the child in your care and pass on to others who will be caring for them, at school or other family members, respite, hospital or clubs.

Sometimes a cry maybe a happy feeling or vice versa but all they can feel or pick up is that there is a surge of strong emotion, a sensation within them as a reaction or response to an experience that they may use that doesn't exactly fit the experience.

It kind of makes sense though, most of us have experienced a joyful feeling and it has resulted in us crying, you know, those happy tears…one minute we are laughing out socks off, the next we are crying—the switch is rather remarkable.

Sometimes this sense can affect emotions and the expression of them by the child not being able to stop crying or laughing easily. It could go on and on, the switch off button can be tricky to find. This is something that can be misinterpreted as being attention demanding or pretending (seen more as a behavioural issue) rather than a sensory one. In fact, many of the sensory experiences can be completely read the wrong way for a large part of an autistic person's life, another excellent reason to closely observe and get to know your sensory sensitive child. What can be interpreted as "bad or rude behaviour" can genuinely be about emotional regulation with regards to this sensory difficulty.

The expression of pain, discomforts as well as the joyful and happy experiences can be learnt by the carer over time. This is an important point, getting to know a person's sensory needs isn't always an easy and obvious process.

Please be kind to yourself, if you are a parent/carer or family member reading this, you are not expected to know everything about your child automatically, no one can, including teachers and other professionals— not even your child. It all takes time for everyone; this is really what my book is highlighting—taking the time to get to know a person is key to being able to help and support them positively.

I am still learning about my son, not only because he is nonspeaking but also because his sensitivity is ever changing as he develops and grows. As he does, he is becoming more experienced in life, therefore he can express some of his discomforts to me in a more precise and accurate way. If I have managed to recognise this in my child, I am certain anybody else can too.

Usually at the beginning of a young autistic child's life, everything is overwhelming for the child and parents/carers. In fact, it can be frantic and chaotic, panic can set in and it can seem that this situation will never change or get easier.

The truth is, it can and it does especially with the early intervention of observing your child closely without necessarily full on interjecting any interference. You will, like I have, start to understand the language your child is speaking through their behaviours and responses to all areas of their environment.

This area of sensory processing, especially the regulation and ability to assess levels of pain and emotional expression can be extra difficult to understand and interpret correctly. I cannot emphasise enough the need to look closely with all that you have to see if your child has any issues in this area. For the reasons I have already touched on with regards to personal safety and the right for them to be able to say no to anything, they do not like or want to take part in, even therapy or play sessions that may look like fun to the outsider.

Often the receiver of any experience isn't the same as what the outsider thinks it is, or how it felt for them.

Helping a child or adult find alternative ways to express their yes's and their no's is both useful and necessary. Methods such as pictures and symbols of a multitude of emotions, AAC devices as well as sign language. Maybe drawing pictures is preferable, sometimes singing songs with specific words are the methods the child has found suits them best. Others may use specific films or favourite TV characters' language to tell you how they are feeling. Whether you are professional at school, a parent or carer, finding imaginative ways to help the child understand language or how to express it is part of your role.

However, if the child is not at a stage where they are able to use any of those forms of communication, the skill of listening and observing, as well as acknowledging their sensory behavioural communication is essential. This tells them they are seen and heard by those who care for them.

I recommend further research into this area of sensory processing, speaking perhaps to Occupational Therapists about sensory assessments along with any advice and knowledge to assist your learning.

Chapter 12
Proprioceptive Sensory System

This sense is fairly unknown in everyday life, unless perhaps you are into fitness and sports this is a word you may have heard before. I admit it was one I did not know about until J came into my life.

For the purpose of this chapter, I will give a brief overall summary of this sense and how it can directly affect an autistic child's everyday life.

The proprioceptive system is located in our muscles and joints. It provides us with a sense of body awareness and detects/controls force and pressure. There is a lot of information online that can be further researched with far more detail.

Proprioception put in a short description is the sense that tells our body where it is in space. Spatial awareness, meaning our bodies' position in relation to the space around us. It is a very important messenger to the brain as it helps us in things such as:

- Self-regulation
- Coordination
- Posture
- Body awareness
- The ability to focus and be present
- Speech

- Space awareness
- Measurement of where our bodies are in relation to an object
- Physical strength—pushing-pulling—picking up and putting down items, including our own bodies., climbing up and down, even walking, hopping, jumping, skipping
- Pressure in touch and small manipulative skills such as writing, drawing, painting, washing and toothbrushing
- Play activities such as catching and throwing beanbags, balls, etc.
- Balance

This is a sense that can severely affect a child's life when at school, nursery, therapy, or other educational environments as well as home and playing outside.

One of the main misinterpretations of behaviours if this is a sensory issue and is not detected, or accepted is the child can be misunderstood for not listening or concentrating when being given instructions. This can result in them being dismissed from class, even school completely because of constant behaviours that are deemed as disruptive.

In intense situations such as school, therapy and home life, this can cause relationship breakdowns and all living and learning environments can become counterproductive for the child.

By you being aware of this sense and its functions, you can detect this as a difficulty for the child or client quickly. This will help massively when understanding the child's physical needs which in turn can help their intellectual and concentration skills.

This can also be a major contribution and reasons for stimming that involve constant movement, as this type of physicality can help stimulate the proprioception sensory system. Further along in the book you will see my chapter on stimming and how it correlates with this sensory function in more detail.

It will discuss how stimming is helping at assisting the child/adult in all manner of ways without limiting them at all. For example, stimming can be used as a tool to assist with focus and concentration. It can also be the key that enables a person to be able to hear what is being spoken or what is going on around them. Less a distraction and more an enhancer of concentration ability.

Once you have read the whole book, the weave I speak of and how connected the sensory systems are and how one area of difficulty can affect another, will become clearer. This is why there are some repeats in my words throughout each chapter, therefore the overlap is easier to see.

Once we know what an issue is, it is easier to see the behaviours portrayed by the child with clarity. What may have previously looked like a mindless physical movement suddenly can be seen as a valid and purposeful act to help them in other ways. (No behaviour is ever mindless, there is always a valid reason)

What may have looked like a child being disruptive in a classroom (for example) because they need to run around the room or climb over chairs and tables can then be recognised as having a need to have the feel of their muscles and joints moving, having some compression on them to find relief (a bit like fidgety legs—restless leg syndrome)—a need that cannot be controlled. Finding a way to be active, will help so that they can become regulated enough to be able to slow the brain and body down together that enables them to focus and take part in a lesson for another 10,15 20 minutes or so. This can also help them at home to be able to relax enough to sleep. Sometimes children with this sensory issue, will need super alert and high levels of exercise just before bed. This is a prime example of doing the opposite to what advice is given to aid a child's sleep.

The usual advice is to put relaxing music on, be quiet and gentle, snuggle down, have a bath, that type of thing. For the child who has proprioception sensory issues that require stimulation in order to regulate enough for them to be able to relax—that routine would be extremely challenging for both child and the confused parents.

This sense can affect the body in a variety of ways which may seem contradictory because on one hand it can affect posture and on the other it can create a need to run and jump, becoming very active and seemingly able in being upright.

Young babies may find sitting or pulling themselves up difficult if they have proprioception issues, it can manifest as them having no energy or not wanting to roll, crawl or stand up and walk. As a child grows, they can be seen as lazy, not wanting to join in with other toddlers who are happily running around endlessly.

On the other hand, this sense when compromised can cause the child to excessively need to run, climb, spin, flap or rock to help stimulate and regulate themselves so their minds can then be calm enough to concentrate on what is being said to them.

The analogy I have already used is like having restless legs, except all over the body. When I get this, I find it very difficult to concentrate on anything I am doing, especially if it involves me having to learn something new, type or listen to someone else talking. The need to relieve the restless feeling in my legs and feet is all consuming disabling me to hear or process anything else that is going on. I have since learnt to deep breath and put my focus on my body and calm it down, although this isn't always successful, sometimes I have to stretch and stretch my legs and arms as well as roll on the floor and sometimes put my feet on very hard things such as stones or rocks.

This sense can affect our cognitive abilities, not because we have an intellectual disability but rather, we have a sensory issue that is distracting our ability to focus.

There is much that can be done to assist a child with proprioception sensory issues. Firstly, I will list some areas on how this sense can affect a young child and adult in everyday life:

- Using a fork or spoon
- Picking up a cup
- Picking up any object however small or light
- Not being able to put anything down unless it is slammed down hard
- Not being able to catch a ball—it slips through the fingers
- Threading beads or doing up buttons on coats
- Tying shoe laces
- Holding a box while someone puts something in it—they will drop it immediately
- Not able to press buttons on toys or pressing extremely hard
- Walking from one end of a room to another over and over again
- Unable to avoid bumping into things or knocking stuff over
- Kicking a ball
- Using a bat to hit a ball
- Brushing teeth
- Combing hair

This list is nowhere near at its end, these are just a few examples to give you an idea of how this sense can affect a person and how.

This sense can affect coordination which is why you will see a baby who is at the early stages of independent feeding, unable to put the spoon directly into their mouths. They will miss and instead get to the eye or ear and wonder why it didn't get to the right place. This is a typical part of developing hand/eye co-ordination skills.

For the child who has proprioception challenges, this can continue into adult life, not mastering self-feeding skills so easily and/or preferring to use their fingers and hands. You see, negotiating an implement is too hard to judge the positioning of the spoon in relation to the food and then into the mouth, all whilst trying to keep the food on the spoon or fork which can be difficult.

It helps us move our tongue as we speak or make sound, it is an amazing internal sensory system responsible for many aspects of our human physicality. If your child is having difficulties with speech or creating full rounded words, this could be a reason why. Being able to move the tongue around the mouth can make a massive difference to how sounds and words are formed.

Breaking the sense and its functions down in this way can help to see how each part of a body may be affected, therefore tools and support can be given as much as possible. For example, if moving the tongue around is lacking when speaking, there may be speech impediments, awareness of this being a sensory issue can help you find the right level of support. An OT (Occupational Therapist) or a SLCT (Speech, Language, Communication Therapist) would be the preferable support for this.

It is important to remember that sometimes there are no cures for such sensory difficulties, but there are things that can be done to ease the grinding or some support with tongue movement in speech, which over a long period of time can help the person to feel more comfortable. (Remember the stepping stone theory? All of this may take time)

Pressure can be hugely affected; this is something my son has challenges with especially on a gross motor element, although his fine manipulative skills are challenged too. He is still learning how to gauge how much pressure to apply when putting things down. He tends to just drop stuff creating a crashing sound as he puts plates and cups in the cupboard. Anything he holds and puts down will look like it is almost being chucked, it isn't he simply finds placing things down gently very difficult. It is an ongoing skill we are working on; we have lost a few plates over the years but the best way for him to be able to gain more control over his movements is practice, positively supporting him whilst he builds his independence and self-help skills.

Below is a list of a few other areas a child may have difficulty in especially when at school or nursery with regards to applying pressure:

- Drawing—using pencils or crayons not knowing how to grip tightly often dropping them or breaking the nib due to too much pressure
- Applying pressure enough to put ink to paper writing very lightly on the page instead or breaking pens due to deep pressure
- Holding a paintbrush and putting paint onto paper—this can be either too lightly or stomping the brush or pen down onto the paper very hard
- Brushing or combing hair can be done too roughly or too lightly no in-between
- Applying pressure in sweeping up or using a dustpan and brush, an impossible task for many with this sensory issue
- Gripping onto a swing or climbing frame
- Jumping on a trampoline—coordination and pressure issues
- Tapping on a keyboard or iPad gently
- Holding onto food laden plates or drink filled cups—likely to drop them
- Not being able to hold a cup and have it filled with fluid without dropping it
- Doing up coat zips, fasteners or buttons on clothes.
- Tying up shoe laces or doing up shoe fastenings
- Washing their hands with soap applying pressure when washing

- Turning on and off taps
- Having buckets filled with anything, and carrying them
- Walking with a box with stuff in, may tilt it or drop it
- Pulling themselves or others from a sitting position
- Doing physical movements such as roly-poly, handstands, etc.

Remember these lists are of examples of some of the ways this sense can affect your child, there will be many other possibilities depending on their persona as well as environments and opportunities they are exposed to.

As pressure is greatly affected it can create problems with having animals as pets. Knowing how gently to stroke a small animal can create problems. Be aware that a hard bash to the animal when you have asked them to gently stroke the cat or rabbit (for example) might happen. This isn't deliberate but another example of a behaviour that can be misinterpreted as being heavy handed or unkind.

You will need to help a child learn this skill by repeating activities and opportunities as often as possible in a contextual manner. Usually whilst a child is naturally playing or engaging in something they are enjoying or like to do. If they love playing in water, you can incorporate some playful activity that involves holding a small bucket while you pour a little bit of water from a height to make it fun, laughter is so important when assisting a child in any skill.

Gross motor coordination is affected with this sense too, which can mean a child may have difficulty in:
- Hopping
- Skipping
- Jumping
- Balancing on a wall or climbing frame
- Ladders on a slide may be tricky so being aware of this for their

safety

- Running fast could be hard especially when there are other children running around with them
- Getting dressed—putting on socks where coordination and pressure is needed in order to put the sock over the foot
- Putting jumpers or t shirts on over the head can be very difficult
- Putting on a coat or cardigan coordinating the correct arm in the right hole
- Brushing teeth for both coordination and pressure appliance
- Eating—preferring to use their fingers and hands to eat as it is easier to navigate without an added implement to have to figure out the weight and size of in relation to food and the body
- Placing objects into places such as cupboards or boxes
- Moving their bodies in dancing or specific movements such as exercise regimes
- Clapping hands
- Doing two things at the same time such as talking and putting stuff away (or two tasks at the same time)
- Batting, kicking, throwing, catching or bouncing a ball
- Knowing how to push or pull a trolley or toy pram
- Roller or ice skate
- Bike ride
- Skateboarding
- Skiing
- Bouncing on a large ball

Again, this list can be endless…this short one gives you an idea of how much a child's life can be affected if this sensory system is needing stimulation or regulation. The list above only shows when the sense is hypo and so such activities may be difficult, however if it is hyper sensitive the opposite can occur where activities such as bouncing on a large ball or trampoline can be sought out and needed in long periods of time, bed times are a great time to engage in these types of activities if the child needs it—they then have a better chance of sleeping.

Both Occupational and Speech and Communication Therapists can really help your child learn more about their body's movements and functions in this area. They can give you some great activities to positively support your child as well as alternative ways to aid self-help skills and strategies.

Eating issues, particularly around chewing and swallowing can be down to this sense. As this sense is also responsible for helping us move our jaws up and down to chew and bite onto food. This means a person with this aspect of difficulty may not be able to chew food very well, or will chew down too hard. Grinding teeth and moving the jaw around can be another physical act that they are compelled to do to get some kind of relief, even though it can be damaging, long term and often painful.

My son is able to chew his food more now he is older, but he still will, if I am not watching to remind him—chew a couple times and then swallow. This means he is swallowing large chunks of bread or meat which can cause him to get discomfort in his chest, (indigestion and clogging) this is an ongoing skill I am helping him with. I constantly remind him to eat slowly and chew more, we also work on having intermittent sips of water to assist the food going down his gullet.

I also make sure that I cut up his food quite small—whilst I am encouraging him to be self-reliant in this area, at the same time I am ensuring he is safe so to not choke on his food. He is also learning how much food to put into his mouth—sometimes he will put almost his whole hand into his mouth full of food, which can create gagging issues. The combination of coordination and applying pressure are present when eating and drinking which he still is figuring out. (I feel that this may have been a major contributing factor why he did not want to eat, when he was a bit younger)

The combination of Occupational Therapist (OT) and Speech and Communication Therapist (SCT) is a good one, particularly with this sensory issue.

This is another of those senses that needs time (often years) for the child to be able to master the right amount of pressure or to be able to coordinate their bodies to where they want them to be or how they wish to move in relation to another object or person, whilst other skills are learnt sooner.

My son has learnt how to pull things that are heavy, he can sweep up using a broom or sweeper. Once he is reminded of the movement and how to coordinate that with his hands and arm, in conjunction with the rest of his body, he is able to do the activity. The more he practised this activity the easier it was for him to remember how to do it. Yet he still needs a little prompt each time, where as in the earlier days of learning this he needed me to spend more time showing him by holding the broom with him.

He is still struggling to put things down gently or apply pressure when using utensils or some machinery. I use these as examples to demonstrate how some skills will be easier to master and others not so much.

Here are some activities that can be fun and playful and positively support proprioception sensory skills:
- Cooking—weighing, measuring, mixing etc. all great coordination skills as well as applying pressure to either build up as practise or to feed the need to hold and mix using their muscles and applying pressure
- Sweeping, vacuuming, mopping (so long as the noises are not too much)
- Climbing stairs and ladders, climbing hills and rocks
- Swimming—jumping against the waves

- Asking to pull you up from the floor, obviously they have to be a bit older and bigger—and you may need to use your own body weight to assist for a while, now my son can fully pull me up from the ground using his hands

- Yoga moves—this is fantastic for coordination and applying pressure on the limbs for certain positions

- Dancing—any silly movements that can create a giggle—building up the moves and mastering them in time—the important part is the movement of the body

- Climbing and crawling using all arms and legs at the same time— this is a great coordination activity as well as applying pressure

- Trampolining—mini ones for indoors can be great for the beginner and those who need to run and jump all over the house—large ones with the safety surround net can be brilliant for enabling them to bounce off the sides to their hearts content

- Bouncy castles—these are robust enough to handle a child who needs that deep pressure to assist them in feeding that sensory input of knowing where they are in the space

- Climbing frames—of all different types—helps with spatial awareness and coordination—be mindful of the heights as some children find it difficult to coordinate themselves back down. When they easily went up—reversing the movements can create a freeze…I have climbed up many a time to rescue my son (when he was younger)

- For the slightly older or more coordinated developed child—using hand tools such as hand-held screw drivers or large paint brushes to paint walls or large pieces of paper

- Pushing and pulling trolleys that are filled with their toys or some food shopping—slowly building up as they develop the skills and build a memory within their bodies system

- Being squeezed (like bear hugged) or having a weighted blanket, being in small spaces, snuggled up tight—this can be very helpful at bed times, either bed tents or weighted blankets (check safety

guidelines for correct weights whilst sleeping)
- Swinging in a cocoon swing for both indoors and outdoors under a weighted blanket can be and feel heavenly!

Another area that can be affected with this sense and spatial awareness is within their visual skills.

Navigating when something is close or far away can be tricky. This means they may put something down too early. For example, placing a cup onto a table but misjudging it and the cup falls to the floor spilling its contents or breaking.

Another example can be when climbing on a large frame—not being able to see the distance of the next bar to step onto it causing accidents.

This can affect their ability to figure out numbers and letters, remembering the order of a word or sentence in either reading or writing it down as well as speaking the words or numbers.

This can cause great challenges in being able to write anything down in a logical order. This is not to be confused with an intellectual disability. It can be extremely frustrating for the child who knows what they want to say or write but cannot because this sense is causing difficulties.

Drawing maybe very difficult too, not the want to do it but the ability to be able to get the hands and eyes to work together to create what they have imagined in their minds eye.

All of these difficulties can create some behaviours from the child that express their frustrations.

- May become disruptive by destroying their work because they cannot do what it is they mean to do.

- They may become withdrawn and not want to take part in any such activities such as drawing or writing—which can cause problems at school especially (This is where using iPads instead of pens and paper make a lot of difference to a child's school day)
- They may be reluctant to go to school or take part in any activities that require coordination and balance and concentration (so quite a lot!)
- They may cry, shout, scream, stim or distract by other means.

If you know your child or the child in your care, whether at home, classroom or the therapy room has proprioception challenges there is much that can be done to help, such as:

- Give them opportunities to move with lots of short breaks during the school day—(this should ideally be child led) you cannot and should not try to control sensory needs
- Let them stand up instead of sitting on a chair
- If they need to stim—do not prevent them from doing so
- If they need to leave the classroom for short periods of time—give them the means to do so and offering a satisfying activity to enable them to regulate—(just standing outside the class will not be helpful)
- Giving them aids to assist with reading and writing—such as letting them use their fingers more than an implement of a pen, etc., such as a touch iPad or use voice activated iPad
- Listen if they say they need to stop doing what they are doing and ask them, 'What do they need?'
- Help them to manage their own time frames of concentration rather than what someone else says is satisfactory
- Include plenty of physical activities that are non-competitive with anyone else as this adds pressure on top of a lot of effort being needed to take part in any activity such as PE
- Activities that promote spatial awareness of their own bodies as

well as other objects (fun and creative activities) this is where OTs can be really helpful (spinning around in a hall with arms out is a great one)

- Avoid using rewards to keep them sitting still, this is something that needs support with and feeding, rather than expecting a young child to control this need for sensory input—treating it as a behaviour that can be controlled can cause bigger issues for the child in aiding the need to move or run even more intense

Of course, as with any sense there are the extreme opposite ends of its abilities. I have spoken a lot about a lack of, there is also a heightened proprioception sense which can enable a person to have brilliant balance and coordination, such as gymnasts and ballet dancers (for example). They may be brilliant at basketball or throwing a netball into its net, they may climb and be brilliant on a will frame—which can almost cause you to worry and then wonder how they do not fall and hurt themselves.

They too may be able to figure out math sums in their heads without the need for writing it down and showing the workings out. They may have excellent writing skills and be competent in using their limbs in ways that may be deemed advanced for their age development.

Additionally, like all the other senses, there may be a mixture of both, where some areas are competent and others not so. There isn't a straight line with any of the sensory processing challenges I have written about in this book, as with autism itself, there isn't a one size fits all. Although autism and sensory processing are stand-alone conditions—they both have vast diversity and uniqueness depending on which human they reside within. There is no one size fits all scenario, all of us are different in every way, we can have similarities of course, yet still be unique in its detail.

The proprioception sense is a complex one and I have only touched the tip of it—further research is needed to fully understand its complexities and possibilities. Speaking with other parents or people who have this challenge is always worth it wisdom. Along with seeking advice from the Occupational therapists who are usually the most knowledgeable about the sensory systems. This chapter offers an introduction to a very complicated and intricate sensory system which can be the key to understanding your child's behaviours.

Chapter 13
Oral/Gustatory,
Taste and Mouth Sensitivity

Sensitivities in this area of the sensory system can affect many aspects of a person's life, which can be quite easy to identify once the child becomes around 2 years old. Younger than that can make it more difficult to notice and therefore go undetected during the child's early months of life.

After all, it is a natural and expected behaviour of babies to put their fingers and hands in their mouth along with anything else they come across. At least, for a short while in their development and discovery stages.

Most babies will automatically put objects into their mouths to investigate it, a natural built in survival mechanism we all have, if it tastes unpleasant or is too hard, the baby knows and will drop it and move onto something else.

However, for the mouth—sensitive, oral seeking child this phase continues into daily behaviour which can last for the lifetime.

This chapter will talk about both mouth and taste sensitivity as well as sensory seeking to appease the need to have something in the mouth for a variety of reasons. Defining what the specific reasons are, can be more difficult to figure out. Why do they need to have something stimulating their mouth all the time? Why does your child repel from having their mouth touched or are unable to eat a variety of food and flavours?

Eating and drinking for oral sensitive children is the most obvious aspect of life that is affected when mouth/taste sensitivities or both is something the child has difficulties with.

I have touched on this a bit in the next chapter which is all about smell. This can create huge worry to parents and carers for very obvious and valid reasons. I would say from experience that 1 out of 3 autistic children have some sensitivity when it comes to either their mouth area or with tasting foods, drink or both.

When my son was a baby, he would enjoy different foods and textures being in his mouth, in fact he would put everything in his mouth (usual and expected behaviour for babies) Yet, with him I could see there was an urgency to it, he seemed to be quite frantic in his quest to find stuff to either rub across his mouth and lips or put in his mouth and eat (more of this later)

Food, for him at this young baby stage was easy, I home cooked all his meals and revelled in the fact that I was providing healthy, home baked wholesome food. A mixture of vegetables and meats, fruit and all manner of textures, he enjoyed dairy too.

He loved to eat multitude of the same thing over and over such as bananas of up to 8 a day. He did this with strawberries and raspberries, devouring pallets of them on a daily basis. He went through a stage where he would eat 12 mini petit pois yoghurts, seeking them out himself by going to the fridge and pointing.

Way back then I hadn't yet realised he was autistic, I just saw a baby enjoying his food and having a healthy appetite, I was so happy as a new mum that food was a joy for him. I accepted his need to eat multitudes of the same thing day in and day out. Lots of young babies and children do the same so I had no reason to suspect anything other than be happy.

Slowly, over time he began to eat less—leaving all the wholesome fruit, vegetables and yoghurts, instead only wanting bread or dry buns, as well as natural foraging foods (more about this later)

He was around 16 months old by now and his pallet had completely changed. I began to worry and started to buy and cook all kinds of different meals, just to get him to eat. It seemed like he had gone from oral seeking to oral avoidance in a few months. He still needed to put non-food stuff in his mouth and rub across his lips but food was suddenly too much, too stimulating, causing him to gag and wretch.

His mouth was now a super sensitive vessel that could only tolerate bland, beige foods, like potato waffles and buns. Sometimes he would eat a veggie finger or a veggie nugget, anything else was a no-no. As he began to develop, his sensory sensitivities became stronger and his awareness of them increased, meaning his mouth area was now unable to cope with most food along with teeth brushing and face washing.

This can happen to autistic children as they grow and develop, in any area of the senses that seem to appear where those sensitivities had not been prevalent before. This is why sometimes it is believed children became autistic, rather than were born autistic.

It is more understood now, that you are autistic from birth, nothing makes you become autistic. While there are many sensory experiences that can create behaviours that can deem appearing more autistic than when they were born (in some cases, not all) and from a quick glance or an untrained eye, this can look like a child has suddenly become autistic.

There is a lot more research evidence on this subject, if you are interested in finding out more, I would suggest you seek out the appropriate sites. Along with speaking with the autistic communities, who will confirm they were born autistic rather than developed it at a later age.

For the next 10 years, he had a very limited diet. Here are a few examples of what his oral sensitivity could allow him to eat:

- Plain toast
- Plain buns/rolls with sesame seeds on
- Potato waffle
- Hula hoop crisps or plain crisps, sometime 4–6 packets in a day
- Only drink water or seek it out in puddles, rain drops or leaves
- Freddo frog chocolate bar
- French fries—plain
- Pepperoni (found by a fluke when his dad was eating one—this was very surprising as they had such a strong flavour but he ate packets of these for a few years)

Within that 10-year period, he would continue to minimise his diet until it was just plain buns, French fries and Freddo chocolate bar. This latter diet lasted for 6 years. It was a worrying time for me I will not lie!

To help boost his vitamin intake I found non-tasting vitamins which cost a lot of money and were not easy to find. Before I found the ones, he couldn't taste I wasted a lot of money on different types, makes, flavours, sprays, capsules and tablets that I crushed into his food. There are more nontasting vitamins available on the market nowadays, although you do need to research carefully and ask specific questions to ensure they are non-tasting and of a good quality.

Each and every day I would prepare him meals that I would leave by his iPad which is where he liked to eat his food. I gave him no pressure, just offered it and every day he would decline.

Then, one day out of the blue, when he was 14 years old, he suddenly started to eat the meals I had prepared for him. It started with him eating some toast one morning before school and that same day he ate his evening meal—he has continued to eat like this at almost 17. He now eats an array of food, including smoked salmon and all kinds of vegetables. I will forever remember the day he started to eat toast and dinners, what a relief.

However, he still has many sensitivities and definite no's, such as: he cannot eat sauces, gravy, diary, egg or slimy food, not even yoghurts, (which when he was younger, he couldn't get enough of). His vegetables are a mixed of raw and cooked, some he can enjoy when cooked but will gag if raw and vice versa. It has taken years to get to understand what he can enjoy and what he cannot. I have always respected his choices (even when I was concerned about his health) forcing him or pressuring him to eat wasn't an option for us.

More importantly to mention is that it has taken him years to figure out what his own sensory needs are in regards to food and texture as well as taste, colour and shape. Whilst we, the parent, carer or therapist is busy finding ways to help and offer suggestions to the child—it is vital that they are given the space and respect to find their own pathways through their sensory systems too.

They are the ones feeling the experiences the environment gives them. They will know how intense something feels as well as how nice it is. As they develop and age, they will be able to understand their bodies and what it needs the more they are supported. Being mindful to not presume to know what is enough or not enough for another person is a skill learnt through patience and observations.

To this day my son loves to cook, at school and at home, it became a big part of the timetabled activities at school a few years ago. He is in a class of 5 other students with a high staff ratio, a specialised school where practical and life skills are just as important as academic achievements.

He loves to prepare all the food, chopping, slicing and mixing with great pleasure—never does he eat any of it, ever since he was about 6 years old, he has not eaten in class at school. Thankfully because he eats a big breakfast and still enjoys fries and buns (on the way home in the car) and eats a HUGE dinner, not eating at school isn't as big a deal as it was when he ate only 1 portion of chips and two buns a day.

We all experience the world in different ways, our taste buds vary, our like and dislikes can be worlds apart. How anyone cannot like chocolate is beyond me! Yet there are many who do not just as I cannot bare the skin on a rice pudding, whilst others seek it out like it is the nectar of a flower as to a bee. We are all unique in our food tastes and textures. Autistic children/adults will have likes and dislikes as well as sensory challenges that can affect their ability to eat, whether they are hungry or not.

There is always a way through that can help an oral sensitive child find foods that they can manage and enjoy. It may not look like what you had envisaged when you first started out as a new parent. They may need food to be the same colour or a particular texture. Maybe the shape makes a difference to their being able to eat.

If the focus is on the sensory aspect of why they cannot eat certain food or drink particular types of liquid you will be able to, more easily find foods that fit your child where they are at, at that time. By breaking down the details of why they cannot eat, you will then be able to find foods that can fit into the categories that they can tolerate. If they can only eat bland tasting food, then you can find it. Or if it is only dry food, they can tolerate—you can accommodate it. Taking tiny steps and working out what works will create a happier relationship with food in the long term and that is always the end goal, the long game.

Like it has with my son, in time things change with more foods becoming easier to eat, there is so much choice out there, eventually finding textured food that feels good and satisfying will become easy. If it is a texture issue (for example) which is a common reason, you will have something to work from. Accepting that a child cannot eat certain foods for a valid reason rather than not because they are being "picky" or "fussy" or because they just want sweeties will also help ease the journey to finding food that can sustain your child's health. There is ALWAYS a reason for resistance to food and drink, figuring it out is the role of the parent, carer or therapist.

Oral sensory difficulties can also mean a child may want to eat and eat and eat, this is nothing to do with hunger, more so to feed the sensory need of the feeling of chewing and swallowing, as well as the pressure in the mouth and on the teeth. This can be a relief in the jaw muscles also with chewy foods or objects that may be sought out around the house.

As with all these sensory issues, you have the two opposite ends needs, hyper and hypo, this is no exception. Initially, this behaviour can easily be misinterpreted as being greedy or being poorly or having worms. (There are other possible health reasons a child eats and eats) a medical check is always recommended to eliminate any hidden issues of that nature.

Some of the possible reasons for wanting to eat excessively, or have something in their mouth all the time are:

- The need to feel a particular texture and NOT the taste, this can include foods and non-foods such as playdough or sand, plastic— anything really

- They may need the crunch or pressure that hard or crunchy foods give
- Soft textures may feel nicer for them or they could be easier to swallow feeling less painful or aggressive as they slide down the throat
- Temperature can play a part only preferring specifically hot or cold
- Sometimes the sensory needs are not about taste at all but about something else entirely such as shape, colour or smell
- The need for resistant giving foods, like rubber—something that creates a satisfying feeling on the jaw and teeth/gums—elastic enough to be springy but still firm
- To give relief from teeth/jaw clenching and grinding

If your child needs to constantly put food in their mouth, regarding this sensory sensitivity, it is usually very little to do with feeling hungry. If this is the case, then finding them foods that are low in sugar is a good idea, this way they do not end up feeling so full up that they become poorly or constipated or gain weight. Plus, it helps keep their teeth healthy.

You can also find non-food stimulating things for them to chew and bite on if it is the jaw and mouth areas that need the stimulation. Further along in this chapter I have listed a few ideas of chewy type stimulants that could replace the food or materials that are not healthy to chew on. Remember the person needing this relief will not necessarily be thinking about safety, therefore helping find alternatives that are safe is required.

If it is the swallowing that feels good for them, then finding low carb, fat and sugar foods would be better for their health and internal bodily functions. This is possible but not always an easy task, so helping them to find other ways to satisfy that need with other non-food related activities would be preferable in the long term. I have also created a list of ideas further along in this chapter.

As I have already mentioned, sometimes it isn't about needing food in the mouth or being hungry, more the sensory need to have stimulation in the mouth area. My son is the same (As am I, I need to feel crunch regularly, I try not to eat crisps(chips) all the time, instead, rice cakes or nuts work for me.). and so, he would seek out metal, wood, plastic, wool, bits of dirt, playdough, material, literally anything he found on the floor he would pop it straight into his mouth, sometimes he would swallow it before I could get to him other times, he would just want to chew it then spit it out. It was extremely difficult to keep a close eye on him at all times to ensure he was safe.

It certainly improved my cleaning skills around the house. Our carpet and floors were pristinely clean!

He loved to rub anything he held across his mouth, sometimes a few times back and forth across his lips. He went through a stage where he would do this with every item he picked up, even large objects like DVDs or books, anything he held was introduced to his lips first. Then if he could fit it into his mouth, it would go in.

Considering how incredibly food averse he became a few years later it was at first confusing to me. But of course, food stuff is a completely different set of taste buds and sensory experiences in comparison to bits of plastic and cardboard etc. As I learnt more about the oral seeking needs, I began to understand the differences I am explaining to you.

Once I became savvy to his deep need for mouth/oral stimulation, I collected all manner of materials and objects to help satisfy his sensory pleasures. This appealed to the nursery nurse in me and I revelled in filling little baskets of trinkets and safe mouth delights for him to indulge in. I let myself get very imaginative collecting materials that had all manner of textures. As long as I made sure they were clean and safe, as well as not too small that he could swallow them, the world was my oyster.

He would get attached to a particular object for a few weeks, sometimes longer—what would seem odd to most, would please him. Random bits of plastic wrapping I would clean and place in his baskets. Lots of different types of material textures of fabric and metals. Soft things, hard things, household utensils, endless hand-held toys and trinkets.

For years, we had boxes of figurines, cars, trains, play people, squidgy balls and toys, fabrics and wrapping material all over the house.

This would extend into nature, he would love to eat leaves, flowers, seeds, nuts, buds anything he could. This was at first very worrying as we didn't know what was safe for him to eat. I knew a few people who were herbalists and foragers in the UK and I was aware that there are many flowers and weeds that were perfectly safe for him to eat. I had to educate myself so we could have a relaxing time whilst out and about on our nature adventures. I bought foraging books with pictures and it didn't take long to get a better idea of what he could safely eat.

This was wonderful, for years, right up until he was about 11, he would forage when we were in nature, even at the beach he would seek out different types of seaweed and devour handfuls of the stuff. We kept a close eye and knew what was safe—he taught us a lot about natural foods actually. He seemed to know what was safe for him, I have no idea how but he did, leaving anything (in nature) that was not edible because it was poisonous. As we researched and studied the wild foods and seaweeds it confirmed that he had a natural knowledge of what was OK to eat. Incredible really, a young boy, instinctively knowing what he could and couldn't eat in the wild.

The added bonus to this revelation was we learnt that there is a lot of vitamins and medicinal properties in most plants and leaves. It was another skill that he taught me that I may never have studied before.

There are lots of autistic children who have a need to have pressure in their mouths, something to chew on and create a deep pressure that feels good. It can give relief and decompress anxiety and help reduce teeth grinding and jaw-clenching acts that once begin are very difficult to get out of the habit of.

Thankfully there is a large array of toys on the market that are safe and durable, that give a brilliant distraction to children and adults who have developed a clenching jaw or teeth grind or any of the other harmful habits such as listed below.

If your child has a deep need to chew or nibble, it is better to give them an array of activities and objects to satisfy that need. If not, what can happen is they will begin to chew their own bodies:

- Chewing the inside of their cheeks
- Biting their lips until very sore and bleeding
- Biting finger nails
- Nibbling their fingers and surrounding skin
- Toe nails and feet skin
- Excessive nose picking
- Biting their arms and fingers
- Chewing on hair

My son can still do some of the above until he is very sore, so I remind him he has chewie's and finger stimulating toys to indulge in. Now he is older he can see that it is less painful for him to chew on chewie's and fiddle with different types of stretchy and squidgy toys rather than bite and chew his own fingers and lips.

This may take a bit of time for your young child to get to grips with, but once they do, they will really enjoy all the satisfying sensory mouth/oral seeking toys you can provide for them.

There are many activities you can offer them that they can indulge their oral seeking pleasures with such as:

- Safe playdough (homemade with less salt) keeping an eye on their digestive systems to monitor how it reacts with their individual systems
- Large threading beads and buttons
- Blowing bubbles—there are many types of blowing activities available (distraction)
- Vibrating toys that they can place on their mouths
- Water play is a great one for those who seek water or liquid in their mouths and throats
- Finger, hand painting or printing (distraction—keep hands busy)
- Button pressing computer games or musical books (distraction)
- Sequin and other sensory materials a child may find satisfying like fake fur or sparkly hanging curtains (distraction)
- Vibrating toothbrushes
- Chewing on their chosen toys as long as they are safe may be what they need to help them not chew the insides of their mouths or grind their teeth

Remember the opposite to this seeking need is to avoid items or specific textures going on in the mouth. This is where listening and watching a child's likes and dislikes in this area are important. Finding what they can handle and how they can handle it is vital to build and maintain trust and self-awareness of their own needs. This can be very difficult if they find the mouth and lip areas sensitive to textures and flavours. Food is an obvious problem, taking time to gently ease a child into foods they can cope with in the long run can help them build on a broader diet. Be mindful this could take years, as it did for my son.

Teeth brushing is another obvious challenge for oversensitive mouth and taste area. As this is an important part of hygiene to ensure a healthy mouth, teeth and gums, it is worth taking time to find ways to get some kind of brushing or cleaning, even if it is minimal to begin with.

My son had many challenges in this area of hygiene. Being in the bath was not a problem, he would be there for hours sometimes. Whilst we topped up the warm water, he would happily play and laugh in water. When it came to brushing teeth, this was a different matter!

This demonstrates a contradiction in sensory needs as I have explained how much he needed to have everything he touched put to his mouth. Yet inside his mouth was a no-no.

I started him on a small cloth as baby toothbrushes were too much for him. Any toothpaste made him gag and wretch, he would cry and resist strongly. Rather than force him to endure the teeth brushing, we worked with him. This took around 7 years of building up to what he uses now, an electric toothbrush with non-tasting toothbrush, as well as a plant-based one.

After the cloth, we moved to cotton buds. We would literally do one tooth and finish before he got upset. I always had the goal in my mind and knew it was worth taking the time to help get him there. We didn't use toothpaste on his teeth until he was 8 years old. We tried every now and then a different type, until one day he was able to cope with the plant-based one. I was so relieved. We went onto using baby toothbrushes which were super soft and took it real slow.

We did this twice a day for years, the fact that he uses an electric brush now with 2 types of toothpaste is incredible and a huge relief. It helps that he doesn't eat sweets or crisps (his choice) and he only drinks water, again his choice.

We were lucky that we had a school dentist who would go to class and work with the students. If they needed to stand up or walk around, he would go with it while he carried out a check-up. He has healthy teeth, thankfully, and now attends the very same dentist, except he now has to go to his surgery. If it came to any actual dentistry work like filling, he may need to be sedated. We will cross that bridge if we come to it, until now we have and are still building up a positive relationship between him, the dentist and the dentist chair.

My top tips for successful toothbrushing are:

- Keep in mind the end result, so do not rush. Building trust is important
- Use different toothpastes until you find the right fit—there are some non-tasting ones available these days which might help
- Try different types of brushes—hard, soft, small, round, square, vibrating, singing, light up, even cotton buds or a small cloth, building up bit by bit
- Try to get water as a natural cleaner if they can tolerate it
- Keep sweet and sugary foods, as well as salty foods, to a minimum until teeth brushing is a regular activity.

There can be many reasons why a child or adult needs oral sensory input throughout their day such as:

- Bored, either there is nothing for them to do or they cannot find anything that is satisfying for them to do
- Stressed—obviously depending on the persons individual circumstances they could be stressed for different reasons—it could be sensory related or work, school, friendships—anything
- Tired—sometimes being tired can be from sensory overwhelm from their days interactions, as can the stress factor—they may not be sleepy tired but more mind and sensory tired—so chewing and

biting can help decompress this as with the stress and can really help rebalance and regulate their systems

- Over stimulated by something, again daily events such as school or an array of sensory overloads that create a surge of energy that they need to get rid of—chewing and biting—clenching the jaw or grinding the teeth can help with that if nothing else is available or they do not want to engage with.

There are other activities that can give relief to an oral sensory seeker that are completely mouth unrelated, such as big physical activities that require pressure to be used from the body. Gross motor activities such as:

- Climbing
- Sliding
- Skipping
- Running
- Jumping
- Pushing and pulling activities and toys like trollies and carts—sweeping
- Bike riding
- Scooters
- Swinging
- Spinning
- Rough and tumble play
- Rolling down hills or on floors
- Carrying heavy objects (age appropriate)
- Digging
- Dancing and shaking—wriggling
- Stamping /stomping
- Weighted blankets
- Being squeezed
- Hanging upside down

- Bouncing on the floor or trampoline
- Shaking their heads

This is a very similar list to the proprioception sense, somehow the deep pressure created by such activities can help ease the need to use their mouths and jaws to find that stabling pressure and relief.

There is a fine line to finding activities that can help full fill the oral sensory need to help eliminate mouth chewing and finger biting and the more harmful and painful strategies—to the child having to rest but still needing to use those more bodily sensory inputs, for they also give a sense of pressure built up release.

As we have learnt throughout this book there are many sensory overloads that can be at play for an autistic child. Whilst some might have one sensory difficulty, others may have a few all at the same time, therefore activities suggested such as climbing, pulling and pushing or playdough, to name a few may create sensory issues in other areas which could prevent them from wanting or being able to indulge in those activities.

There is a range of the oral sensitivities and needs a person may have throughout their life. Circumstances can alter the need to stimulate the mouth area, such as:

- Puberty creating surges of unusual feelings internally that create a need to chew or bite (like a stim)
- Feeling poorly, headaches, toothaches, earaches, upset tums, anything that they may not be able to cope with so the need to bite and nibble eases distracts or acts as a counteractive pain, like a diversion
- Puberty stages that create physical changes in the body—bodily hair, developing breasts etc. can all play a part in the need to up

the oral stimulation

- Events that happen in a day either at school or something they have seen or read online that have caused distress or sadness
- Excess of energy that they cannot rid themselves of any other way because of different sensory or physical limitations
- Because it feels good to them in some way or another—until it doesn't! like if they get too sore or start to bleed, if fingers nails are bitten down to the bone (for example), sometimes it does get quite extreme
- They haven't figured out another way of getting the sensory input, pleasure or release
- A multitude of emotions such as feeling scared, anxious, excited, happy, bored, frustrated, angry or tired
- The environment they are in is unpleasant to them, a specific place—maybe it is filled with unhappy memories, maybe it is too noisy or busy, bright, hot, cold…
- A specific person creates uncomfortable feelings for a multitude of reasons both positive and negative whether it is because the environment is stressful or calming or the child is bored, unhappy or overwhelmed.

This is why a one size fits all approach will have its limitations and failings for the person needing the support. A multitude of sensory challenges for an individual can create huge problems, such as when some of the solutions for one sensory need can be helpful, they can be counterproductive to the other senses. Learning about your child/client and what their individual needs are right from the early ages can create a more specific and tailored approach.

All of the above are suggestions and an introduction to the types of things you may observe through your child/client's life. No two children who are having oral sensitivity are going to need the exact same remedies and activities to help them feel better.

Sometimes asking a child to completely give up their preferred tactic, such as finger biting can be too tall an order. I found that it was easier for my son to accept new strategies if they were introduced slowly, whilst still accepting he would need to continue with the current ones, like a slow phase out.

A slow transitional process with an end intention. Stepping stones, sometimes by pushing too hard creates a natural resistance that becomes counterproductive.

I had in the past, tended to panic, especially when he was getting big nosebleeds numerous times a day, through his need to pick and poke. Reacting from that point meant he became stressed and of course needed to pick even more to help calm himself down.

The long game is more often than not the most beneficial in the end. Results that mean your child is no longer getting sore, bleeding fingers, or nose bleeds—whatever the harmful behaviours resulted in whilst helping them find different solutions. As they develop and mature, they will be able to find alternative activities for themselves, or with less resistance to anyone else's suggestions. They would have learnt from experience that some changes can be positive for them. As long as there is an alternative replacement.

I have also learnt that I have to step back from certain things, like nail biting (for example) my son still needs to bite his nails, they get sore and he blows on them. He can feel the pain, more now he is older and he stops for a while. This is when he can begin picking his toenails or clench his jaw, until his fingers have healed a bit then he is back on them. I wish he wouldn't, but I cannot make him stop. He has alternatives to try and prefers to bite his fingernails.

The key here throughout the book is to help your child see there are different options and a multitude of ways a person can be assisted with their sensory challenges. Offering them out, but at the same time accepting they may choose to not use them immediately. Instead of panicking that they may never find solutions that can help ease any distress, give them time to adjust to the new ideas and ways of doing things. Sometimes these new ideas can take a while, maybe days, weeks and sometimes even years before the child can allow themselves to use them. This is the case, especially if there is a deep need for routine (which is my son 100%)

Every aspect of a sensory sensitive child is intense and all consuming, one can affect the other and on and on…so what might seem like a really good idea from your perspective could be a very scary prospect to them.

This is an example of what oral sensitivity can look like, how it can change from seeking out tastes, textures and stimulation on and in the mouth to not wanting or being able to tolerate much at all.

As you can see, oral sensory sensitivities can have many attributes to it, that look like contradictions to the observer. The truth is that most sensory challenges are complex. This chapter has touched on some of those contradictions and opposites.

Chapter 14
The Smell Sense Olfactory

This can be one of the most difficult senses to detect in young autistic children, mostly due to the physical behaviours that can manifest if this is a sense that is highly or under attuned.

As you read further into the chapter you will see the type of behaviours that can manifest because of an overwhelming sense of smell and why such behaviours can be mistaken for health and 'challenging' behavioural issues. Additionally, I will discuss the under attuned smell and how this can affect a person in daily life.

When a behaviour is completely misinterpreted, in this scenario specifically, mainly because nobody has any idea what is going on, huge problems can occur for the child and their relationships with others. As you read on this the reasons will become clear.

Smelling is something that we all do without giving any thought to its functioning ability, unless of course we either lose the ability to smell or if a smell is so pungent it stirs other feelings such as a gag reflex in our bodies.

The most common reason the smell detector may change is when we develop a cold or illness that causes the nose to be blocked or we develop an infected throat. A respiratory issue can cause a loss of smell, although usually temporarily, bringing huge relief once it does return so that normal (for the individual) life can begin again.

Most of us have experienced this in a life time so can first hand empathise on how this can be challenging or at the very least inhibit our eating experiences and pleasures—sometimes both a loss and enhancement of the smell sense can affect ones want to eat, even if they feel hungry.

Imagine having a hypersensitive smell so strong that it causes you to vomit or gag? This can be a reality for the extremely sensitive olfactory sense in young autistic children and adults. Or the other end of the spectrum you have a hyposensitive sense that means you are unable to smell foods that can usually tempt you into eating, stirring up the other neurons that tell you the food is yummy and you are ready to eat/drink?

It can be that those who have temporarily lost their sense of smell have lost weight because they have not wanted to eat as much as they usually would.

I have a very sensitive sense of smell; it took me years to figure out why I would sometimes get tense or agitated or suddenly feel nauseous or giddy. It didn't occur to me that it could affect my moods and ability to concentrate or function comfortably.

I, like many others can associate a memory from a smell that may cross my path out of the blue. Suddenly I am taken to a memory that I may not have thought of for years, this can lead me down a route of reminiscing. It can feel like I am back having that experience again.

Some of these can be very happy memories, whilst others can be unpleasant. Sometimes these memories that are ignited by a smell have led me away from my present moment for a few minutes, to an hour or longer. As I have become older, I have learnt to manage it better, so I can have the memory then come back to the current moment, leaving any of the feelings associated with the smell in the past.

As a younger person this was more difficult for me to do. If a smell hit me and triggered a memory good or bad, I would trail off into a daydream like state and feel all the emotions associated with that memory.

This can happen for children who are triggered as I was through a smell who sometimes are unable to remove themselves from the memory straight away. It can bring up feelings of that experience so powerful that they may become upset or start to laugh, depending on the experience of that smell or they may change their behaviours that can, to the observer look completely out of the blue and be totally unrelated to their current environment.

Sometimes the memory can cause the person to re-enact the experience which can look very odd from the observer's perspective, especially when they have no idea that they are remembering something from a past experience.

For an observer such as a parent, carer or professional to figure out that a memory of smell has caused the change in behaviours (a want to suddenly eat a particular food, for example) will be almost impossible unless the child can express this and explain what is happening. (This can happen with any of the senses actually; suddenly a memory will be regenerated, triggered by something that may not be obvious to the observer.)

As with the other senses I remind you, parent/carer/therapist, to be kind to yourself—you may not get it right straight away, you probably won't. Which is why observing and listening to all of the child's communications, physical, vocal, emotional and behavioural will help you translate what is actually going on more easily over time.

Having awareness of the many possibilities that may be causing the sudden outbursts of behaviours can be enough to get you on the right track. You can then begin to tick them off one by one in your mind once you know for sure if it is a smell or sound (for example) issue.

The sense of smell is a powerful and necessary tool we have to help us navigate our way through life. It can be both pleasurable and pungent smells that help us know when we are unsafe or safe as well as helping us know what we do and do not like. It is a super sense that acts like an antenna—giving us some pre warning of what is happening or what we are entering into.

Many smells can be distracting almost instantly whether they are pleasurable or not. I live rurally and muck spreading happens a few times a year on the fields that surround us.

Sometimes this is an extremely unpleasant experience for me, it affects my eyes, my taste and can also give me a tummy and throat ache, usually a headache because the smell is pungent to me. I can feel quite unwell. The smell can be so intense that I may continue to smell it even when I am well away from the actual smell. It is like it can linger within my nostril walls and it can be very uncomfortable, affecting every aspect of my life until I am released from the smell.

I do not know many people who like the smell of muck spreading but not everyone finds it as disgusting as I do, or has any of the other symptoms that I have.

This is a reminder that we can all smell the same things yet be affected differently. What may not be an uncomfortable or intense experience for you could be the opposite for your sensitive child. Please never assume or underestimate the distress some sensory experiences can cause for many autistic children and adults.

As an adult I can express my discomfort and remove myself from an uncomfortable environment without having to explain myself to others. A young child cannot, especially if they are non-speaking and have not yet found a way to communicate their feelings, other than through their behaviours. Sometimes the younger child will not have yet figured out (like me) that it is a smell that is causing them to feel overwhelmed in some way.

Here is a list of some of the behaviours you might see an autistic, hyper smell sensitive child portray—as well as some places they may not want to go to because of the smell:

- Itching or rubbing their noses excessively
- Sneezing a lot
- Hitting themselves in the face
- Head banging
- Screaming
- Running around
- Reluctance to enter a room or a building
- Tiredness
- Anxiety
- Reluctance to play with some creative play such as play dough
- Reluctance to eat or be in a kitchen
- Reluctance to be around animals especially in zoos, farms or in their own homes
- Avoidance of close contact because of perfumes, deodorants and shampoo smells on another person
- Avoidance of food to eat or drink
- Avoidance of some clothing especially new ones with packaging smells on

- Detergent and washing powders on clothing causing a dislike of clothing
- Displeasure of a bubble bath or shower due to smells of shampoos and soaps etc.
- Avoidance of teeth cleaning
- Being outside in nature due to the many natural smells such as animals or muck spreading or harvesting time
- Vomiting
- Sticking items up their nose/nose picking—nose bleeds/sores
- Nose snorting

Here is a list of some activities they may not want to engage in because they have a hypersensitive sense of smell:

- playdough
- painting
- bubbles
- cooking/baking
- Soft play centres—for the restaurants, smelly feet odours! And sweat
- zoos and farms
- some houses of relatives or friends (every house has smells) even if it is pleasant to you
- kitchens
- bathrooms—bath times
- eating and drinking
- school eating halls
- children's parties
- swimming pools
- hospitals/dentists/doctors
- Being close to people because of perfumes and hairsprays etc.
- dogs/cats/pets in general

- shops of any kind as well as cafes
- markets
- cars
- petrol stations
- seaside

A lot of the physical behaviours and bodily reactions to smell such as vomiting can be a build-up of being in smell for a long length of time. Strong smells can cause headaches, stinging eyes, itchy/tingling noses, coughs, itching, rashes and an unpleasant taste in the mouth.

There could be other symptoms that can go unnoticed in an individual for a while and then suddenly what seems to be out of nowhere to the observer the child may vomit, or start to cough repeatedly. When they have in fact been suffering unbeknown to anyone else because they are not having the same smell intensity experience as the child. You cannot be aware of something you do not feel yourself; it takes practise and patience to learn all of these signs and possibilities.

This list could go on and on as smell is everywhere, depending on your child/adult and their sensitivity, anything can smell unpleasant to an individual. A particular building can smell, I remember my primary school story time carpet stank really bad—which made sitting on it extremely unpleasant for me. Story time was one of my favourite activities so I found a way to endure it, which was usually sucking my thumb and placing my finger inside my nose holes.

I also recall going into some people's houses when I was a child and the smell of the home was unpleasant or really strong, the feeling it gave me was often a foreboding one, I dreaded going into the house. This had nothing to do with the people in the house, more often I really liked them but the smell would somehow create a fearful feeling inside of me that I could not explain. Most of the time I would suffer it, stay quiet, very quiet—silent, thumb in mouth, squash my nose entrance and hope we would be out of there as soon as possible.

Entering buildings where medical appointments or assessments take place, which is more likely in a hospital or medical centre where there are many strong cleaning product smells can be extremely difficult. The smell plus the added unknown of what it is can create a lot of fear and anxiety. This can be enough to create a complete stand-off, or shut down to not want to enter that building, or if they have entered then began to be affected by the pungent smells, doing everything they can to escape.

Imagine feeling a smell inside your nose and throat intensely—yet not knowing or understanding what it is. All you know is you feel completely overwhelmed with physical symptoms that you feel the need to run in the other direction.

Hospitals do smell, as soon as you walk inside one it hits you with a mixture of detergents, bleach, antiseptics, food, numerous human odours as well as medical equipment and endless plastics. This can be a valid reason why a child may not want to enter a medical building. To this day I have to take a breath and mindfully prepare myself for the smell intensity if I ever enter a hospital building.

The very nature of living life in any environment means there are going to be smells, everywhere, home, nursery, school, even places where a person's favourite activities take place. Although being in nature is seen as a lovely and healthy activity, the smells can be constant depending on the season and the environment, enough to stop a smell sensitive child from wanting to be outside in certain environments. Flowers and shrubs, even trees can smell awful to a sensitive person. The lovely smell of a flower maybe so strong that it becomes horrible, not the smell but the intensity of it.

Keeping your own home neutrally smell free can be a near impossible task. However, it can make a huge difference to a sensitive person. If you can eliminate the ones that cause the most discomfort, life can become much easier for the child.

As a smell sensitive person, I can categorically say that hyper smell causes extreme behaviours that are all consuming in everyday life. It is made easier for me now because I am responsible for myself and can create environments that have as little (unpleasant) smell as possible. I can express my needs and dislikes and find strategies such as covering my nose, holding my breath or simply leaving an environment or staying away from a person if their perfume or deodorants are too pungent for me to cope with.

Children do not have this strategy, at least until they can either use verbal expression that is understood by the adults around them or have other forms of communication available that enable them to explain their difficulties.

If I was experiencing some of the many intense and unpleasant smells that I do and not be able to leave or minimise the impact it has on me, I am certain I would go into a hyper ventilated episode. It has happened to me numerous times in my life where I have almost passed out, vomited or cried, mostly become anxious, shaking as well as headaches and tummy aches.

Most of us wear body odour deodorants, perfumes, shampoo and use detergents that make our clothes smell nice and fresh, we have flowers in the house and food cooking. Some homes have candles burning that have pungent smells and plug in air fresheners. (One of my worst.)

Schools have many cleaning products and soaps available at all times and some equipment such as pens and markers can have a very strong smell. All of this can add to a child's distress which will affect their ability to concentrate, communicate, interact and be happy.

As with some of the other senses, this one can affect a child's want to take part in certain activities. It may not mean they do not want to do the activity itself, but it is the smell of certain equipment, environments or the person who is offering the activity that has a smell too strong to cope with that stops the child from wanting to take part.

Imagine being hungry and needing to eat but not being able to because of the smells of a kitchen or food cooking? On top of that not being able to express why you feel so anxious or have behaviours that are deemed as "bad" or "disruptive" simply because those around you are not aware that you are experiencing a smell overload.

I know from life experiences that most humans veer away from unpleasant smells as quickly as possible. We express ourselves very loudly either by vocally saying how awful a smell is or by physically covering our noses or walking, even running away.

I have seen adults coughing, eyes watering and a rapid need to escape and once they have, they immediately resume a calm and happy state. It's as quick as that! So, if a child who is smell sensitive is suffering unbeknown to anyone who is caring for them, these kinds of behaviours can increase in intensity developing into full blown meltdowns which can result sometimes in misunderstood presumptions and unfortunately, punishments.

Being told you are disruptive or "naughty" can be soul destroying for the child, creating anxiety and fear of going anywhere because they know they will not be understood.

A child might try to run away from a situation, let's say a school dining room or an art lesson because of the smell of paint or clay (for example) and not being able to say what is going on? Eventually this creates all sorts of problems that can affect every aspect of a person's life and, if it is school that is problematic, their education also.

Schools and nursery settings can be very smelly places, I know I was a nursery nurse for 28 years! Although for many the smells are unaffecting negatively but for those who are super sensitive, as I have already said, even a nice smell can become unpleasant. Think of a smell you really like, imagine that it is turned up by 100% I can assure you it wouldn't be such a nice experience then!

So, how can you help support a child who has this sensitivity?

The obvious way is by removing any smells that cause them distress, some of which are possible, but many are not. This is when it can be tricky, yet not entirely impossible.

The key is to figure out if they have smell sensitivity to begin with and the best way to do that is to observe their behaviours and interactions and reactions to their environments.

When it is possible and if the child can communicate with you what is happening for them, ask questions and help them found solutions together.

If they cannot yet communicate in any way, it is up to you to provide many forms of communication tools, such as pictures and photos of items and food stuff, use Makaton sign language or introduce an AAC device that can help express what is going on for them, draw pictures if you need to.

If you know that smell is an issue, you can eliminate many excessive ones from the home and replace with less intrusive smells such as:

- non smelling detergents
- non smelling hair shampoo
- non smelling soap and bubble bath
- non smelling toothpaste
- do not use smelly candles or carpet cleaners
- allow them to eat away from a kitchen, even if the eating table is there, they will not eat if the smell is too intense
- Give them foods that you know they can tolerate—they will not eat if they cannot bare the smell—neither would anyone!
- Avoid activities that are smelly such as zoos and petting farms etc.
- If they can handle, wearing a scarf across their faces to cover the nose for certain situations that could be helpful
- Find alternatives to play materials that are non-smelling for example homemade playdough is almost smell free compared to the shop bought type. Or if there is a smell, they like such as almond or peppermint (examples) you can add a few drops in the mixture.
- If you can avoid them going into hospital buildings or doctors do—I have managed this with my son for years, by explaining to the doctors the situation. There are always other ways they can be supported medically either by zoom or video footage or photographs of any cuts or issues.
- Accept any reluctance to take part in activities that may seem "fun" to you or the other children (remember they may want to be able to take part but cannot cope with the smells)
- Place a dab of essential oil of a smell you know they like either on a cloth hanker chief or directly onto their skin (check that this is safe to do so first) just under their nose or even on their top

Obviously, there are times when it is impossible to avoid such situations and with all the will in the world some experiences are to be endured.

It is better to know the reasons why your child or a client may be having a tough time and expressing themselves in some of the ways I have listed. Even if you cannot avoid a hospital visit or treatment (for example) you can minimise it by using some of the suggestions I have offered, or come up with your own distractions. (Although this may not always be enough.) You can talk to them about their feelings and validate them.

For the person experiencing any kind of sensory overload—it is made worse when nobody understands why or has any awareness of how they are feeling. Even if there isn't a solution, having someone understand the reasons will make a huge difference. This means you can become a better advocate for them—asking others to make accommodations to help soothe your child's sensory needs.

If a behaviour, for example is hitting themselves in the face and screaming or maybe trying to run away from a particular room or cafeteria at school—but the reason is unknown, it is assumed as being attention seeking or disruptive. This can result in the child being punished for having an intense sensory, painful experience which is no fault of their own.

Being misunderstood and wrongly reprimanded for how you feel when you cannot do anything about it will begin to create other problems for the child.

This is a theme that runs deep with many autistic and sensory sensitive children and adults. So many misdiagnosed or undiagnosed cases of children who have intense difficulties in a multitude of senses. All of which can be put down to "bad behaviour" because the causes are unknown, solutions cannot be made and so the behaviours increase or multiply and the child becomes isolated further. They can develop trust issues and emotional depressions as well as low self-esteem. Anxiety related health issues grow and communications break down completely leaving everyone feeling totally defeated.

This is another example of why the most important and beneficial outcome for everyone is to find out and learn about sensory processing difficulties as early as possible. Although sensory processing difficulties are not the reasons for all behaviours, it does affect a massive amount of an autistic person's life, especially when younger. Knowing what those sensory challenges are cannot solve every issue or difficulty. However, it can and will for many and at the very least help to minimise the unpleasant effects it can have for the individual.

If you do not know how to help the child, maybe by knowing the reasons you will have an accepting attitude that can enable the child to find their own solutions. Such as my son using his fingers to control the input of the sound entering his ear canal, like I have learnt to do, you will be able to support their choices if they choose to not take part in a particular activity.

Hyposensitivity can cause problems too, in ways that can be very harmful.

As we know some smells are there to tell us something is infected, off or dangerous, such as gas, petrol or poisons. If food is off or contaminated, we can usually smell it, this can save our lives and at the very least prevent us from getting food poisoning or becoming intoxicated with a dangerous gas.

If a child is unable to smell such smells, they can continue to eat contaminated foods or walk into dangerous situations without having those natural sensory warnings that help us make a different life or death decision. Usually, a pungent smell will be a warning that even a young child can detect and move away from it (although not always)

A child may not be able to smell poo or find the smell unpleasant enough to not want to play or smear it everywhere. It has been known for children with sensory issues to smear poo and eat it in some cases. This may not just be because a sense of smell is lacking there are other reasons this happens but it is certainly a possible factor.

Another smell aspect for sensitive children and adults can be that a smell is so pleasant that they seek them out.

Have you ever heard of a pregnant person needing to smell a particular substance or item during their pregnancy? Usually, they would not need or even like the smell they suddenly find themselves yearning for. When they do find it, they feel satisfied somehow, it calms them down not knowing why but needing it just the same.

Something happens during pregnancy that creates our usual sensory pathways to either heighten or be dampened down, for most of us it is temporary. Unfortunately for many autistic smell sensitive people it lasts a lifetime.

The smell of bread can be an extremely pleasant experience for people and when they do get to smell it, they go all swoony and feel happy, even hungry suddenly—which can lure them into buying and eating it. Some people have bought bread-making machines purely to experience the smell of fresh bread in their homes.

In some cases, extreme smell (for the individual) can cause people to go into a seizure, although this can be rare it is still something worth mentioning because within the autistic realms it isn't as unusual as one may think. It can start with passing out or fainting, which can turn into a seizure. In fact, seizures can happen with any overloaded sense and I have seen it for myself and heard of it happening, particularly in the smell and sound sensitive person.

Maybe it is more common in this sense because it is the hardest to fathom that it is actually a problem for an individual. Therefore, they are exposed to smelly environments for longer periods of time without anyone picking up on the pre seizure signs.

For example, my son can get triggered by overheating in or out of water, this is a well-known fact and anyone who cares for him is informed of this. Therefore, he is monitored closely and overheating is avoided therefore the likelihood of a seizure happening is very low to non-existent. I knew of a young man who would seizure if he was exposed to sudden loud noises, especially if he could not see where the sound was coming from.

If the condition is not known, pre-warning signs will get missed resulting in extreme circumstances which can leave everyone confused as to what is causing the seizures or fainting, often putting it down to a tummy bug or another physical illness.

Some of the most common physical reactions of an intense smell is to vomit or gag. Obviously if this happens at school or nursery and the real reason is unknown, it will be treated as a suspected tummy bug. The child will be sent home for at least 48 hours as is the common rule under those circumstances.

As I have suggested previously, it is a good idea to get a child medically checked out to ensure they do not have any infections or stomach problems. Once you are satisfied that they are healthy, you can look at sensory possibilities. This will help the teachers and staff create a plan that can support the child's needs. Together, as a team you will find some solutions to avoid specific activities so that your child doesn't have to go through the trauma of the smell inducing nausea and be constantly sent home for 48 hours, which can be very disrupting to their school routines.

Food and eating can be hugely affected if smell is a sensitivity for a person. If we do not like the smell of something, we will not eat it, it goes hand in hand—it would be illogical to eat something we do not like the smell of.

If I am offered something to eat that I have not eaten before, I always smell it. I do the same with drinks. In fact, I smell most things before anything else, not just food!

Food can be a very tricky part of any child's life. So many tastes, textures and smells to deal with, for most children their pallets are limited and need time to strengthen and become able to cope with the many strong flavours and smells on offer.

For the smell sensitive child food, eating and drinking times can be an absolute dread. This can and does create huge problems for the child and a great deal of worry for parents and carers.

As food can be a stressful experience for many (not all) autistic children it is worth spending time on finding out why. One of those reasons could be the enhanced smell sense that is causing them to flee from the very mention of dinner or breakfast time!

When we smell food cooking, most of us react with excitement if we find the smell pleasant, our mouths begin to water and our tummies even rumble. We can become impatient because the smell of the food cooking is luring us in. The same happens when we smell something cooking that is gross to us, we will definitely not be wanting to eat it, no matter how hungry we feel.

It is probably an inbuilt alarm system that says "these smells awful—could be poisonous" perhaps! I haven't researched this to be scientifically factual but it makes sense to me.

Most children autistic or neurotypical can find food with its many flavours and smells challenging. When we are babies just starting out on liquid foods, if we do not like something we will just spit it out, pull some funny faces or throw it back up. This is accepted as a dislike and the parent/carer will offer them something different, no questions asked.

If it was a smell that caused the baby to spit it out, we probably wouldn't know, because the baby cannot tell us at that point. As they grow and begin to use their hands and arms to push away the incoming spoonful of food, it could be the smell that is the driving force. Once again, they may not yet be able to tell an adult that because they are developmentally unable or do not have the language skills to express with.

Most of us probably do not consider that it could be a smell that is preventing a young baby or toddler to not want to eat something. It is usually considered to be the taste that is causing the refusal.

For the autistic, smell sensitive child this can be, as I am sure you can imagine very distressing. Dreading every mealtime, unable to express why you cannot eat and nobody understanding, yet insisting you eat something!

It's the number 1 panic button for most parents, if a child does not eat, worry sets in, for obvious reasons. There is a lot of expectation and pressure on ensuring children eat a healthy and balanced meal. For a lot of autistic children at some point in their lives, this is not a reality. In the end, it can come down to them eating something, anything just as long as they eat.

There have been suggestions made to parents that their autistic children will not starve themselves, once hungry enough they will eat. Well, while this may be true for some, for the many this is not. I have heard story after story of autistic children ending up in hospital because they have not eaten after 5—10 days even though they are starving.

The sensory overloads are so powerful and all consuming that it does prevent an extremely starving child from eating or drinking, this may sound over the top, but it is something that has happened to lots of children and adults.

This is another subject that could have its own book, let alone a chapter or two. There are so many reasons for an autistic child or adult to have issues around food. Smell is definitely one of the top reasons and realities for autistic people.

This can include food environments, such as cafes, restaurants, hotels, cafeterias in supermarkets, play centres, home kitchens, shopping centres and street side burger bars. Anywhere there is food being prepared and cooked.

Sometimes the experiences of unpleasant smells around food can be so bad that just seeing a food place from a distance can create anxiety and avoidant behaviours.

For a young child, both home and school are usually the two most frequented places in their lives. This can cause huge problems.

School dinner halls can have intense smells that linger not only at the actual meal times but also while the food is being prepared and long after it has finished. I can recall the halls smelling of food anytime we went in it to do other non-meal time related activities. Remember my smell is extremely sensitive so whilst the other children and adults were unaffected, I was having a very different experience.

Some classes have their lunches eaten in their classrooms. This can be difficult for the child because there is no escape from the smells that creep out of the lunch boxes and trollies.

A way around the smell for those at school can be to let the child eat their lunch in the classroom to avoid the hall and kitchen areas, but if the classroom is where meals are eaten this is not so easy. Alternative places are required so that the child can eat something without being under enormous pressure, dealing with an overload of smells which can affect their ability to eat their own food.

Managing smells within your own home can be difficult, living in small environments where smell travels around the whole home, or if the kitchen is open planned. Finding a solace place for your child to be to avoid smells whilst cooking is an obvious solution.

Once it has been realised that smell is an issue for your child you can begin to eliminate smells as much as possible. I do not pretend that this is an easy issue to conquer, cooking dinner is a daily occurrence at home with other members of the family to consider. Knowing that this is an issue for a child can be enough to help find alternative places for them to be while cooking tea. For example, if they take themselves to their bedroom and want to stay there for the rest of the day or night—knowing why will mean you can accept this without worrying about them being isolated. If they feel better being out of the smell environment, they will feel much happier and settled doing their own thing than having to suffer unpleasant smell sensations.

Finding food they can eat can take time too, but there are usually some that can be enjoyed by a smell sensitive child. Once you know this is an issue, you can experiment with different types of food and eventually find ones that can make up a decent meal. The most important thing is that they eat something. As they grow and develop many smells they dislike will change over time. This is, like all the other sense sensitivities, an ever-evolving experience.

The key is that the more you can honour and accommodate their sensitives when they are young, the easier life will be for them to function in other areas of their life.

Sometimes offering raw food can be a solution, some foods smell and taste less when they are raw, some do not which is why experimenting with both cooked and raw foods is a good idea.

My son can eat a mixture of both now, some food he cannot eat when they are cooked but loves to eat them raw. If smell sensitivity is affecting their eating habits, this will have a huge impact on their mental health as well as their physical health. Living under constant stress of sensory overload on top of being hungry will mean the child is unable to show their true personalities. When anyone is under stress, they behave differently to their natural state.

It is totally possible for an extremely sensitive autistic child to live life with a calmness to it, finding ways to eliminate their sensory pain is key to their peace.

For some autistic smell sensitive children as they grow and develop the intensity of smell enhancement decreases, like it has for me. Although I do still have extremely sensitive smell, I have also developed a tolerance for some smells that once drove me crazy, many smells I can now happily experience without gagging or feeling headachy and dizzy. This is different for everyone, but what may seem like a lot when your children are young, does not always mean it will be that way for the rest of their lives.

I know I have mentioned this in almost every chapter, I do because it is a point worth reiterating. The earlier their needs are catered for, the easier it may be to support them in learning and discovering their own body's needs, enabling them to naturally develop healthy strategies to cope and manage their own sensory requirements. Each day is a learning opportunity for you as their carer and the child/adult for themselves. Some will naturally dwindle away whilst new ones may arise but with your support and encouragement in honouring their choices, they can find ways to manage it without having to live in constant stress.

This strategy is a win-win in any situation. If your child is going to need 24-hour care for their entire lives, your close observation discoveries will be passed onto the carers they meet throughout their lives. You are ensuring they are cared for and honoured when they are living away from home. If they can live semi- or wholly independent, you have supported them in being able to advocate for themselves confidently—which will hopefully save them from having to mask their truth where ever or whomever they meet throughout their lives.

Chapter 15
The Vestibular Sensory System

The vestibular sensory system is a strong brain stem sensation that requires a lot of effort to calm it down or awaken it. When it is over responsive it needs a lot of input to help regulate it, just as it does when it is under responsive. It seeks equilibrium within the body and if for some reason that is compromised, all sorts of physical and emotional problems can happen.

It is a sense that is located in the inner ear that helps us feel balanced, it also supports the movement of our head and controls muscle tone. If this is out of kilter in either an over or under responsive way, it can interrupt the sense of feeling safe, particularly from falling over. Creating a vertigo sensation if the sense is over responsive even when standing on 1 or 2 steps, or standing upright.

This is an internal sense of our system that acts like a compass for the body and its movement in relation to the space around us. If out of balance, the compass needle spins around aimlessly causing all sorts of problems and physical sensations that can make it very difficult to function in life.

This is another of the senses that I did not know that much about until I met my son. I was familiar with the word but had never given it any thought to what it was responsible for and how intensely it can affect a person's life, especially when there are interruptions to its function.

I suggest you continue to research this sensory system for a deeper understanding. Scientific explanations along with details about the intricacies of its function and exact location are abundant online, there is much to learn about it.

During this chapter just as I have with the others, I will give you examples of how this sense can interfere in a child's life if it is over or under responsive—in a practical way. There will be examples of activities to offer to help support their individual needs which can be easily provided whether at school, home or work.

Most of us have experienced an earache at some point in our lives, we have been spun around and know what the feeling of giddiness is. The strange experience of not being able to anchor yourself to something solid without having to fall to the ground.

As a temporary feeling it can be funny—many games at parties are of being spun around—the aim of the game is to see who can stand the longest. It's impossible to keep standing or keep your head upright whilst feeling giddy, resulting in you falling over without any control over it at all.

Another feeling of giddy is the fairground ride, you lose all sense of where you are in space, the spinning is so fast that you cannot make sense of anything. Most of the time this feeling lasts for a short while and we return to a normal balance.

When our vestibular system is over responsive, the feeling of giddiness is apparent most of the time—it does not take much for us to feel disoriented and giddy from the simplest of activities.

When we get giddy or feel we are about to fall, it creates a panic within our bodies that says we are in danger. That usually encourages us to hold onto something (for example) or to sit down or leave the current situation you are in. This gives us a reassurance that we cannot fall, it is an automatic response that happens instinctively. Typically, many of us only experience this on a few occasions within our lifetime.

Some of us find being on a boat easy, no sickness at all. Others will feel giddy and become very nauseous, that is all part of our vestibular system doing its best to keep us stable and depending on whether our bodies are slightly under or over responsive will determine how we can get our "sea legs" and remain balanced without the feeling of falling or disorientation.

Living with an over responsive vestibular system, can be a life in a constant fear state—having that feeling that you may fall over. This can create extreme adrenalin and cortisol rushes within the body that has a huge impact on a person's ability to think rationally and logically. Focus can be affected and therefore behaviours can appear irrational and out of context.

The whole point of the body releasing those two chemicals is to get you to move as quickly possible away from the situation that tells the body there is danger, whilst running away or using physical exertion to remove yourself or protect yourself from the danger the adrenalin and cortisol is used up. Then the body can regulate itself again to create a calmness within you once again.

By being in a constant state of flight or flight, the body has to use its adrenal glands a lot, creating the chemicals, yet not finding the peace it needs to restore and rebalance. This is why it can create other issues physically and emotionally for the child who is living with this over responsive sense.

Here is a list of some activities a child may find uncomfortable or frightening and will do their best to avoid them, or will show strong resistance to, most certainly not enjoy:

- Running
- Walking
- Hopping
- Skipping
- Rolling
- Dancing
- Car journeys
- Bike rides
- Train and bus rides
- Horse riding (especially fast, like a trot or canter)
- Being held upside down
- Being in crowded places with lot of people moving about
- Watching spinning visuals on a TV or computer screen
- Being spun around in any way
- Stairs and escalators
- Going to a park because the swings and slides, see saws create dizziness and nausea
- Going up ladders
- Being held up high
- Being on a boat
- Walking on bridges

If a child has an under active vestibular system, they may seek out such activities or feel the need to:

- Spin constantly without getting giddy
- Rocking—either sat on a chair or just using their bodies
- Swaying
- May be fidgety and restless

- May shake their heads from side to side
- Run
- Jump—on or off anything they can
- Climb and roll down hills or around a room
- Want to sit in a swing for long periods of time
- Stay on a trampoline and not want to get off
- Seek out weighted covers, like a blanket or other objects
- Hang upside or sit on the sofa upside down
- They may head bang or slap themselves around the face
- Run around in circles
- Bike riding fast
- Really enjoy horse riding or fairground rides to the point of sleeping

As you can see from both of the lists, they are full of play activities that most children are exposed to. It is easy to then see how a child can miss out on lots of fun activities because of a fear of losing themselves within the activity where they longer feel their own bodies as well as feeling all the symptoms I have listed above.

Some of these activities can be dangerous to begin with for the child who seeks them out and they will act frantic as they run or spin. It isn't until they get that satisfied feeling of being balanced, solid where they can feel their bodies' movement in space that they then can calm down and feel at peace.

This may last a couple of hours or as little as 30 minutes, and they need to seek more spinning or running (for example) to regain the calmness.

This is a difficult feeling to explain to someone if it is lacking, most young children will not know why they need to spin or run frantically around a room, they will just do it in response to their natural bodies' messages that seek out this sensation.

Children who have this strong need to move, wherever they are can appear hyper active. (Of course, there are other reasons a child may run and climb fast and enthusiastically for ages around a classroom or home.)

If a child is showing you that they have to keep moving or have a need to hang upside down or spin, are jumping on and off sofas or stairs at home, giving them safe alternatives is going to help them find that peace they seek.

There are many activities you can offer to a child within your home however small or big it is, both inside and out:

- Swings for indoors or outside
- Hammocks are great too
- Spinning toys that you can sit or stand on—there are many on the market these days
- Dancing opportunities
- Yoga moves that move the head around in different positions are very good
- Monkey bars
- Head stands
- Kids aerobics
- Bike riding
- Skate boarding
- Surfing—body boarding
- Skating
- Running games
- Horse riding
- Spinning on foot
- Being swung around by their legs held under their arm pits (with their permission)

Think about a young child in a classroom at school who has this sensory need which they have no control of. Offering behavioural rewards such as sticker charts or treats will not work, for this is not a behavioural act. In fact, using rewards to keep still for a certain length of time (for example) will only create bigger anxiety and frustrations for the child as they will now have the sadness that they continue to fail in reaching the goal to receive a prize or a sticker.

Displeasing the teacher and being constantly told off or removed from a classroom and then further expected to sit in an office or isolated space will cause bigger issues and relationship breakdowns. Some children can end up being expelled from schools and nurseries because the teachers are unable to cope with the constant need to move or fidget.

Once this has been identified as a sensory need, practices can be put into place to support the child when at school. Having that sensory assessment with an OT, that I have spoken of, will help pin point exactly what it is the child needs to help re balance them to a peaceful state. This can then go into an IEP (Individual Educational Plan) or a PBP (Positive Behaviour Plan) (*I personally do not like the latter term, however it is used in various Education and therapy sessions, so I am making you aware of such terminology*) so that the support workers and parents/carers can create a programme of activities that will enable the child to move when <u>they </u>feel the need to.

By making small changes to the day, that enable the children to move around the classroom whilst having the lesson, or run around outside for more regular sessions you will support this area of sensory stimulation need.

Something as simple as standing up instead of sitting down could make all the difference. Having short intermittent breaks where everyone (if they want to) can stand up and shake their bodies or run around the classroom pretending to be aeroplane's (or something else) can create fun and exercise especially when the children are under 10 years old.

It is important to highlight that this should not be adult led scheduled. Setting specific times when a child can run or jump etc. can be counterproductive if the child isn't ready for that exertion. It can lead to them becoming confused about their body's messages. Remember the intention is to enable the child to be able self-monitor when they need certain activities or releases, changes—whatever it may be to help bring them into a more peaceful state. No one else can truly know when that is required for an individual. Your role as carer, teacher, therapist is to recognise and accept this is a sensory need. You then create space or allowance for the person to act, whenever they feel the need to.

These suggestions might seem radical and disruptive to have in a classroom at school but the positive effects, outweigh the negative ones, tenfold.

Many children miss out on an education because their behaviour isn't understood or there aren't the resources (support staff) to assist them through no fault of the teachers and LSA (Learning Support Assistants). If you can pinpoint this as an issue early on, a sensory assessment can be carried out by the OT and a diagnosis can be confirmed this means you can have a reinforced tool to get the ILP created as soon as possible. I want to add that you do not need an official diagnosis of sensory processing disorder to warrant creating an IEP with any activities to support a child's sensory needs.

Everyone benefits, especially the children in the class, because some of the suggested activities can be incorporated into daily lessons for everyone to enjoy.

Inclusion for all children to be in a mainstream setting has to surely include the individual needs of the children met so that they can thrive regardless of their neurodiversity?

Earlier on I touched on the point that an over responsive vestibular sense can create a fearful feeling in a child. I want to explore the extreme measures a child can go to because they are in this state of flight or flight when experiencing this over responsive internal sense.

Many of the activities I listed (and please remember there will be many more that the individual person will find terrifying that I have not included) will be what are typically fun for a child to engage in. This is another example of accepting when a child says they do not want to take part in an activity. There will be a valid reason, figuring out what that is will be key to supporting them and finding solutions or alternative activities they can enjoy.

Presuming that a child will want to go jump on a trampoline (for example) or learn how to ride a bike because "it's what children do" could be a major mishap if the child in question is experiencing vestibular overdrive.

Imagine how you feel when you are scared, what happens to your body internally and externally? Perhaps you can feel your heart beating faster than usual and very loudly. You may find yourself breathless and unable to talk clearly. Sometimes palms can become sweaty, even the whole body can get very hot.

When fear really sets in, especially when it is the kind that we haven't figured out why we are scared, it creates irrational behaviours and thinking. For example, when something makes a noise when you are in the house alone, or perhaps you are out walking in the dark and you hear a sound you cannot locate, the unknowing is what initially creates instant fear. All your natural defence systems start to kick in, adrenalin and cortisol releases, narrowing your mind and logical thinking to a linear thought of safety first, think later. Either get ready to fight for your life or run as fast as you can to get out of that situation.

With all of that in mind, it isn't so hard to understand a child's behaviours when faced with the activities suggested if they cannot bear to take part in.

Below is a list some of the possible behaviours that indicate the child telling you they do not want to take part and just how much they mean it:

- Verbally saying "no, I don't want to, I do not like it or I can't" words to that effect
- Closing their eyes tight
- Hitting themselves or if being carried or held, hitting out at others in a distressed way
- Screaming
- Shouting
- Running away
- Laughing (this can be a nervous response to something stressful) which can be misleading to the observer until they know the child well enough that it is something they do when scared or in pain
- Falling to the ground and crying, screaming, kicking, hitting
- Vomit or soil themselves—remember this is a fearful feeling of flight or flight so depending on the extremes of their fear this can be a reality
- Passing out/fainting
- Going into seizure
- Stimming more than usual
- Go into shutdown (they do not move from where they are) for a long period of time
- Trembling
- Spitting
- Various vocal ticks and sounds

Some of those that are listed will look like what is described as a meltdown, which can happen for endless reasons for any individual experiencing overloads of sensory systems across the whole range.

Some of these reactions can look surprising and unnecessary to the observer. The response may not warrant such extreme behaviours to a person who has no idea what is going on for the child internally or why they fear such activities that everyone else is loving.

This is why this sense is described as a strong stem sense which does require a lot of stimulation when under responsive or creates a lot of fear when over responsive. The research on this is intensive and thorough these days, so you can find out in much detail to enhance your understanding of this sensory system.

When the feeling of falling is primarily present in a child most of the time, just by simply standing up and walking around (for example) life could be, for them a very challenging experience. This is intensified when you feel deeply a threat of having to get on a swing or trampoline, any activity you know will increase your feeling of deep fear and panic, even though you do not understand why.

Yes, such behaviours look extreme to the observer, because that is how it feels to the child—it feels extreme, intense, overwhelming, terrifying and life threatening. The chemicals in the body are overtaking reason and rationality so any words of comfort or encouragement will most likely go unheard.

Processing language and words when in such a fearful state is almost impossible which can mean the child will continue to do whatever they need to do to let everyone know they are feeling scared. This will not include listening to any words of comfort or instruction by others, this doesn't mean they are being dismissive or rude.

Feeling out of balance and afraid on a regular basis can be exhausting. Eventually the body has to rest and get some respite from the constant fight or flight responses.

Some children and adults who experience this as a sensory issue will need time and space to recuperate and restore. This might be a few hours in a day or it can be as long as a week.

Some children may feel poorly on a regular basis, headaches, tummy aches, nausea or sickness. They may get intermittent mutism or a need to sleep or shut themselves away in their room. They may not want to eat or drink very much or be near anyone for hugs and reassurance.

For others, they may want to be hugged and squeezed and reassured, remember there are no hard rules for a one size fits all. These are examples of what can happen to one extreme to the other so that you can get a loose idea of what an over or under responsive vestibular sense can feel and be like for someone.

In previous chapters, I have mentioned that sometimes the activities on offer are not the issue. More the feelings that happen when engaging in them which can be just as disappointing for the child or adult as it is for anyone else. Not being able to take part in an activity they may really be interested in because a sense is too over responsive or limits their ability to engage in it can be confusing, as well as upsetting and frustrating. Particularly for a younger person who has not yet figured out why they feel the way they do.

An example of this is something my son has dealt with his whole life. You have read how his auditory sense is over responsive, he has, over the years found his own way of managing the input of sound that enters his ear canal. For years, he did not take part in activities, instead watching others play and engage while he sat at a distance to reduce the extreme pain and noise he was experiencing. As he self-discovered to place his fingers onto the entrance of his ears he could begin to engage in some of the activities he was interested in.

One of those is swimming as he adores the water, the most recent one is carpentry. He absolutely loves to create with wood with the support of his class teacher and his support companion during the school holidays. He has become a brilliant apprentice in this activity, which is such a joy to witness. Sometimes he can wear ear defenders, others he cannot, which does limit his skills with certain tools because he needs to hold one of his ears to reduce any noise from either the tool he is using or for the instructions being given at close proximity.

For years, he would watch, wanting (unbeknown to the observer, carer, teacher, me!) that he really wanted to be able to participate in some activities he had happily sat away from and observed. He just hadn't found a way of easing the sound input that was comfortable for him. (He does also genuinely like to watch others having fun)

Now, at almost 17 he does take part in carpentry—he has made all types of things from plant holders to cat shaped calendars, even novelty sheep foot rests! He uses tools such as hand drills, sanders and saws, he bangs nails in, which makes a huge racket. He has now adapted another way of reducing sound into his ear canal by using his shoulder top to press against his ear. Sometimes he just takes a breath and gets on with it, needing short breaks throughout the activity so he can get a bit of a gap between intense noise.

To see him do his best to overcome his discomfort so that he can take part in his much-loved activity is wonderful. It is also humbling (for me) I know how much a big deal it is for him to almost sacrifice his comfort so that he can enjoy his much-loved activities. We are constantly working on ways to help him be more comfortable around loud noises whilst supporting him in his choices and needs.

J never does anything he does not want to; we have raised him to be able to clearly express his likes and dislikes by accepting them from birth. This has reinforced his own abilities to know what he can enjoy and what he wants to try. When he was younger, he was not able to do such activities, now he has had more self-experience, knows he is in control and is respected he can positively engage in more activities than ever before.

It is also worth reminding you that watching and not participating is a joyful experience for some people, never needing to engage with the other children, getting their fun from seeing others having fun. Watching is a brilliant way of learning the rules, and how an activity is done. Observational learning is a skill I advocate throughout this entire book, not just for adults to children but for anyone wanting to learn about something.

Have an open mind to all possibilities when observing a child's behaviour through the sensory lens, closely focusing on their communications in behaviours. The language being spoken through their sensory reactions and interactions can be the key to your understanding more clearly what they are telling you. After time, you can begin to learn when it is the discomfort that is preventing them from taking part in a specific activity, rather than the dislike of the activity itself.

For the under responsive vestibular system, the opposite behaviours can be present in the child to those of an over responsive system.

You may find that the child, especially when young   will   look tired or unmotivated, they may not be running around using all that energy a toddler often has. They may appear agitated and teary; they may be unable to concentrate or focus on any one thing and be restless but not know how to ease the uncomfortable feelings.

Some children are unable to nap during the day because they are too fidgety however sleepy they may be. They may have restless legs or arms, this can be confusing to the carer, parent as the child will be tired and need sleep but just cannot lay still enough to doze off.

We all know what it feels like to be over tired and not be able to sleep, it can create all kinds of funky behaviours and agitations that make for a challenging time.

Another aspect of being unable to sleep is a busy mind. This can create an overwhelm of thoughts and experiences that have happened during a day. Sometimes the child/adult will be thinking/worrying about the day ahead, whilst in bed, as well as all the stuff that happened that day. This can create some issues in a busy household, where the rest of the family sleep easily and the busy mind child is finding this time of the night very difficult.

When it is quiet, everywhere else the brain will be freer to go over and assess the day's events—the good—not so good. Sending a child to bed early to get to sleep could be counterproductive. Anxiety builds up, along with other symptoms such as restless legs and the mind gets busier. If a child has not learnt or is unable to learn strategies that can help to calm them—this can feel torturous.

Finding tools that can assist your child to relax—even if they cannot sleep is a huge relief. This may mean they need a variety of things to help the relaxation to set in, such as:

- Some type of music that they like in their headset or turned down low (it might need to be loud and not what you regard as relaxing music; remember it is their choice)

- Audio books
- Projectors of sea or calming lights (depending on your child's visual needs, some need bright some may need pastel)
- A blast of exertion in a big way just before bed—remember the (proprioception sense needs stimulation to be able to relax, as would the vestibular)
- Epsom salt bath—has magnesium and is great for relaxing muscles (research it for more detailed info)
- Allow them to have a low light on if needed
- Accept they may not be able to go to bed at a typical time for their age
- Weighted blankets in bed (or a heavier duvet, as there are safety regulations and advice on whether weighted blankets are safe for sleep time)
- Having their bed on the ground—this can help enormously—feeling closer to the earth, somehow can make a difference.
- Sleeping with a pet—if they have a close relationship with them, a dog or cat can help reduce anxieties
- Deep massage (if they like the pressure) including the head area if they can tolerate it, especially if they ask for it
- Allowing them to have their iPad—if they cannot sleep, they will feel more rested if they can have something to help keep their busy brains from going into overload
- Writing or drawing the things they did that day (they may not want to talk about it)
- Using a particular colour night light. There is research into which colours can help soothe. For those who need a stim to relax them, it may be a different colour

There are many things that can be tried if your child has busy mind. It could take a while before the right thing for them is found, I hope some of the ideas above can help you think outside the box of "usual bed time expectations".

This is why an OT (occupational therapist) can be a great resource in this department. They can pinpoint the issues early on and so can help you find activities that can encourage the child to become more active. This will help activate their vestibular responses which will help them feel more balanced.

Once the child has started to engage in more physical activities you may find they will be wanting them all of the time. My list above shows some of those examples of not wanting to come off a trampoline or scooter (for example)

They may want or need to keep hanging upside down on some monkey bars or sit upside down on the sofa…jump and jump and jump. This is a very strong stem sense so it will need a lot of stimulation to activate an under responsive system—hence the continuing need to want to jump and bounce or run and run!

Once there has been a perfect balance found for the child, they will begin to self-regulate and manage their own needs far more efficiently than when they are slightly younger or are experiencing this sensation for the first couple of years.

For most children in any under or over responsive sensory system, they find their own equilibrium state and what were maybe repetitive activities when younger, they become less so when they get older. Not because the sensory need isn't there anymore but because they have found ways to keep them in a more balance state. An adult has the freedom to make their own choices, at their own pace. Children have adults guiding their activities, including when to start and stop them.

If a person with a deep sensory need to run, stretch, spin, climb or jump is told to stop before, they have reached that balanced state, continuous frustration within their body's will endure. It will look like, (to the adult) that the child/adult is never satisfied or calm. Whereas if they are supported in bouncing (or whatever it, is they need) to do for as long as they need it, eventually the need was decrease. It won't disappear completely, it was, however become less because the body (sense) will be getting what it needs when it is needed.

Allowing the child to feed their needs in all senses will help them to regulate more easily for themselves for the rest of their lives. This is the long-term goal, is it not? Self-reliance and knowledge to know when they are beginning to feel overwhelmed (for example) rather than have to live in a constant state of overwhelm or under whelm because they had not been given the time and space to discover what is going on in their bodies and to give their bodies what it is they need.

Chapter 16
The Importance of Repetitive Activities

When you think about it, most humans have repetitive and daily activities that become patterns of behaviours. This is considered to be an acceptable part of life without any cause for concerns. It definitely isn't seen as "obsessive, inappropriate or a problem".

This, however has historically been a cause for concern when it comes to autistic children and adults.

Seeing routines as a usual and perfectly acceptable part of their day is frequently seen as an issue. Restrictions and rules are suggested by numerous therapy strategies, particularly behavioural driven ones. For the autistic child, their needs of repetition are often labelled as unhealthy and possibly developmentally dangerous. It isn't uncommon to see assessments and reports written describing repetition as "obsessive behaviours".

It is important to see the need for repetition from your child's perspective because they are necessary for your child to thrive. This chapter will hopefully help you understand why.

The word obsessive automatically creates a negative mindset, it is deemed a bad thing to be obsessed with something, rather than see it called a favourite thing to do or an enjoyable game, within the autistic realms it gets labelled OBSESSIVE. This almost always implies a problem that needs to be stopped. There are numerous reasonings and theories behind this attitude. The most common one is the belief that they will not want to play or engage with anything else and it will keep them "locked in a world where they cannot engage with others".

Whilst this may be true for a while (not the locked away in another world part, but the want to play with one specific toy/activity for long periods of time, days, weeks, even years), it will not be that way forever. In all the years I have been a mum to an autistic son, met and engaged with 100s of autistic people as well as speak with parents about their child's experiences, never has a child got stuck forever on one thing.

Like all children, they grow and develop and gain a sense of themselves, this is a necessary part of that natural process. Meeting the needs of their sensory input and output, is an integral part of their self-exploration, remember your children are figuring out about themselves just as much as you are.

They do this, (we all do) with our environments and what is directly around us, whether that be nature, toys, people, food, animals, furniture anything! Once they have saturated themselves with a particular activity and then eventually feel the need met, naturally they begin to reduce the amount of time they spend on that one activity, they will move onto something else. Their interest in different things happen, they might need to be similar—they might not, but they do change.

They may continue to go back to their favourite past time whilst spreading their interests to other things. This isn't necessarily a regression, more an anchor point, a familiar experience that they feel safe and happy in. For some, it is because it is a joy and that is that. We all have favourite pastimes, don't we? Sometimes we do not do a particular activity for months, maybe years, then find ourselves wanting to go back and play with that old toy or game just for the joy and memory of its pleasure.

There really isn't any need to panic or presume that your child will only ever want to spin (for example) or watch a particular film or TV show forever. Like I have said, even if they do, they will most certainly find different interests in time that replace or are an addition. If they do continue to want to watch the same movie over and over for years, is it really a problem or cause for concern?

The problem with having language written into an assessment for a diagnosis such as "obsessive and inappropriate" is that recommendations are written into a statement of needs or in an IEP (individual educational plan), ILP (individual learning plan) or BDP (behavioural development plan.) the other problem with such language is that it can become normalised as acceptable to state all repetition is damaging or limiting to the child's learning and development. When in fact it is the total opposite to that. The benefits are huge.

Right from the get go when researching how to get a diagnosis you will find the familiar descriptions using language with those familiar words, obsessive, another is "age inappropriate" which can very quickly become accepted as facts by parents and professionals who are working and living with autistic people.

The repetitive behaviour becomes something to fear and eradicate without considering what goodness and enrichment it gives to the actual autistic person. There is always an enormous array of valid reasons that are particular to the child or adult.

By learning, understanding and accommodating repetition behaviours and activities you can advocate positively and confidently for your child throughout their school lives. This will in turn inspire others to follow suit. This is a time now to get into the modern mindset of supporting and accepting autistic individuals from their perspectives. Doing this means challenging old systems, method and assessment programmes which does include the language used to describe and label autistic behaviours and their reasons.

We all need to be seen in our individuality and autistic people are no exception!

This is a part you can play in this much-needed change—there are other, parents/carer and professionals who, wish for the old systems to change and new language to be used so that autistic children and adults can be positively understood and accepted in every way.

I think it was Buddha who said there are many pathways to enlightenment. Well, there are also many pathways to living life and thriving. Being autistic and sensory sensitive are two of those many pathways, just as valid, as important and intelligent as any other…

Some therapy programmes such as behavioural modification therapy will focus on any repetitive behaviours and work on reducing them. This suits the needs of the therapist and what they deem as appropriate and healthy. The child's needs are least looked at and sometimes the reasons why the child is needing to repeat activities aren't explored.

When you are new to parenting, having had no experience with child development on top of knowing nothing about autism this can take you down a path that speaks in very restrictive terms. Hearing and reading such words early on can be the beginning of a mindset which can lead you to feel afraid for your child.

Parents can feel isolated and separated almost immediately because their autistic child's repetitive behaviours are painted to be mind boggling and weird. The urgency to stop repetition and instead overflow the child with a vast variety of activities to prevent repetition from developing.

As soon as a repetitive behaviour begins panic sets in and the need to stop it becomes the goal. This can be detrimental to your child's development, growth and happiness. It can get in the way of their learning on many levels. By stopping such behaviours without understanding why they are doing them will also prevent you from learning about and getting to know your child, how their brains work, what their sensory needs are and how they feel when they are left to indulge in their favourite activities.

If there isn't a safety issue around the choices your child makes then there really isn't a need to feel worried about repetition.

Before I go any further, have a think about what your rituals are, what kind of morning routine do you have? Do you need to drink a certain drink made in a particular way? Do you have an order that you like to have your morning routine in, EVERY day?

My bet is that you do, for many things. Even occasional events like going on holiday or the movies. Wearing the same familiar types of clothing or using the same sun cream, having to buy popcorn and a hotdog because that's what you do when you go to the cinema! (Just an example.) These are all ritualist routines.

We have all experienced a routine or a familiar event in our life, not happening for one reason or another and it throws us off for a while. You can usually get over it eventually, the point I am making is to remember that uneasy feeling you have when a routine you like is changed. Look into the uncertainty you feel, even if it is a tiny amount. It is still a feeling of short-term panic or your brain scrambling to find an alternative way to help get your mind focused and your feet on the ground again. It might make you feel irritated, anxious, frustrated? Take a bit of time now, if you can to think about this truthfully.

It is also easier to remember when you have full control over your life because you are an adult, even neurotypical children (as they become older) get to have some choices and make decisions of their own likes and dislikes. In fact, it is encouraged, well, routines are a part of that.

Sometimes when we are rushing around trying to get ready for work or some event and something in our usual routine goes array it causes some of those feelings of frustration.

Most of us have repetitive behaviours without thinking about it, even if it's watching a particular TV programme every day at the same time. Having the same meal on a particular day of the week or a meal with particular food types that you have to have with it. Maybe you like wearing the same brand of deodorant or makeup. Do you have a Sunday routine that is the same every time? Perhaps you enjoy a particular radio programme, TV show, pop star?

Most of us find change difficult, in varying degrees, look at this last couple of years. Huge changes have taken place on an almost daily basis. This has created feelings such as uncertainty, anxiety, instability not knowing what to expect or how to behave or feel about things.

For some of us, this has triggered the need to find stability in other ways, establish new routines and activities. The truth is we regroup and create more routines and rituals that can help create a feeling of safety, calmness, perhaps peace of mind, stimulation of mind, distractions? Some of those routine activities will help you sleep more easily, feel less stressed out, and instead centred once again, maybe you feel in control again— most certainly relaxed.

Since reading the previous chapters on the senses and their many challenges for autistic people (children in particular) it is easier to see why repetitive play is an important part of their daily life. My intention is to help paint a bigger picture that enable you to see why routines and repetition is a necessary tool in learning about the world around them in a joyful and meaningful way. Most importantly they can learn about themselves.

ALL children repeat activities, how many do you know who are neurotypical who watch the same TV shows or movies over and over again, for years? This is usually seen as completely acceptable in a young child's life—however, for the autistic child, red flags are put up as a major problem that needs to be challenged.

I decided that this topic merited having a chapter of its own because not only is it a massive part of autistic children and adults' lives—but also because it causes so much stigma and displaced concerns. (This attitude is beginning to wear down, but it is still around in some camps of therapy and out of date attitudes, so look out for it.)

A lot of time is spent worrying about a child only wanting to do one activity or watch a specific movie over and over again, when in fact it is a completely usual part of a child's development and joy experience.

Some professionals (not all) will suggest that repetitive play should be minimised in order to get your child to cope with change. It is also seen as a negative behaviour and a reason why a child may not socialise with their peers or family. I have already mentioned the too, common phrase of "being locked in their own world" therefore the goal is to unlock them from some kind of prison it is presumed they are trapped inside of.

Autistic children are not locked in their own world—they are as much a part of the same world as any other human. Their focus is on other things for completely valid reasons, which I am hoping will become clear throughout this book, most of this is due to the intense sensory processing reasons you have already read. In this chapter, I aim to give you some more insight into why repetitive play is important and necessary for your child and, particularly why stopping it can create more harm than good.

I have stated that children develop as they grow and age, all children do, some do it at different stages and in different ways, this includes repetitive activities.

Young babies of any neurotype are given activities that are repeated, never is this seen as a problem; in fact, it is encouraged by professionals to help familiarise your baby with people and their environment.

Repetitiveness is seen as a positive way of educating a baby and toddler in every way, it is recommended as the most advantageous way of helping a baby learn and develop.

During specific developmental stages it is suggested by "child care experts" that you offer your baby/toddler a more diverse array of toys and experiences.

For neurotypical children, this usually happens naturally, an inquisitiveness arrives, an enquiring mind and off they go exploring every nook and cranny of any environment you put them in. Having to need eyes at the back of your head to ensure they are safe as they innocently and enthusiastically discover the world.

For the autistic child, this can be the opposite, instead they need a smaller choice of interests. There are many reasons for this depending on the child's sensory, cognitive and physical needs, abilities and experiences.

As they grow and develop further, the child's interests can become smaller again, finding favourite things to do and engage with, TV shows, creative activities, certain toys and games, clothes they like to wear can all become repetitious. For the neurotypical child, this is not considered a problem. I am not suggesting it should be, more so the opposite. Why then is it regarded as a problem for an autistic child of the same ages?

You have already read and discovered in this book that sensory processing for an autistic child is incredibly intense which is one of the main reasons why repetitive play and interaction is necessary. In fact, it doesn't feel like repetitiveness and it never gets boring or invaluable to the child who needs it. Joy is found every time the activity is experienced just as much as when it happened the first time—the 1000th time is equally as much fun or as comforting and beneficial—this is a very important point to remember, their personal tireless need to have it will show you the importance of enabling them to continue with it.

Keeping their world smaller means their stresses and energy is kept to a manageable level for themselves. Although for many autistic children this isn't the reason, or the only reason they do it. They are simply living their life in the way they choose without worry or need to move onto something else.

How do you cope when you feel overwhelmed? How do you manage your day when you are feeling under par, ill or anxious? Usually cancelling appointments, minimising interaction with others as much as possible is the first thing we look to do. We seek comfort, veering towards our favourite activities which calm us and help us feel nurtured and relaxed.

Why would autistic children be any different? Their experience of the world is far more intense and confusing. We already know that sensory processing consumes every part of their life, so perhaps needing more isolated time with what they find comforting and joyful is beneficial in more ways than has historically been realised.

Seeing repetitive play as a problem has previously (throughout history) been the opinion of many professional fields. This attitude showed a lack of understanding and knowledge of autism in general terms. Today we are becoming wiser in the old beliefs, particularly in autism.

Here are just a few examples of activities/experiences your autistic child may need to have repeated the same every time:

- wearing the same clothes
- wearing the same clothes for specific activities
- wearing the same shoes, slippers, trainers
- wearing specific footwear for specific activities
- eating the same foods, eating in the same order at the same time
- Drinking the same drink every day, at the same time—in the same cup
- Toys—wanting to play with the same toy over and over, needing to take it everywhere they go
- Needing toys to be put away in a certain place in order
- Wanting to watch the same movie or TV programme over and over, numerous times a day whilst still getting as much joy from it as the last one
- Games on the computer—same as the TV—never tiring of replaying the same part of the game over and over
- Blankets and bedding—needing to have the same every night including the same colour and textures
- Teddies and soft toys
- People—doing the same types of activities with particular people and no one else
- Wanting to go to the same park on the same swing (for example)

This list is not exhaustive there will be many more as each autistic person is different and will need consistency and repetitive activities for different reasons.

Here are some possible reasons to get you into the mindset of perhaps why a child needs repetitive activities:

- Gives calmness and peace—shutting out all other stimuli
- They have sounds, smells, colours, shapes, sensations in an order that they can expect without any surprises—anything different takes a lot of effort to process.
- When watching movies on repeat voices have the exact same sound, pitch, tone, phrasing, time phase without any changes at all, unlike a human voice.
- They may experience certain feelings and sensations within their bodies that make them feel happy or good when hearing the voices and seeing the shapes, patterns and characters of the show.
- Some (movies and characters) can help them understand concepts of human relationships and social rules which is easier to process and understand instead of real humans who have constant differing delivery.
- Being surrounded by neurotypical people can be a complicated experience when trying to figure out or even notice nuances, body language and social cues
- They enjoy the activity a lot!
- It is their favourite thing just for the joy of it.
- All of these seemingly tiny changes can be huge and exhausting to your child, having such finely tuned senses means you notice the most subtle of changes in a voice.
- Watching familiar movies or TV programmes can help them to figure out their own experiences throughout their day at school perhaps or at home.
- They are learning about colours, shapes, language, numbers (depending on the activity)

- Repetitive play creates a safe place, familiarity feels good to all of us especially when overwhelmed.
- It is a peaceful and calm place for your child. The environment and daily life have huge demands on the senses as you have learnt so wanting some sameness is completely understandable.
- What may seem like a boring way of living, watching the same DVD or listening to the same phrases over and over again isn't for your child. They find constant joy in re visiting the same activities—this is a beautiful attribute.
- Repetitiveness means your child can rest. They know what is coming, not having to concentrate and feel a vast array of attacks on the senses.
- They are learning about themselves and how to self-regulate—a skill they will need all of their lives.
- They are learning many concepts depending on the activities they are re visiting.
- Physical activities on repeat can be what keeps them regulated (for example) needing to bounce or spin, run or jump, being squeezed or have heavy weights on them may help them know where they start and end in relation to space. (Vestibular and proprioception senses)
- Repeating activities can be a coping mechanism for the rest of their day. Without them they may shutdown, meltdown or mask how they really feel, which would ultimately result in them shutting down completely unable to engage with anyone.
- It is their right to do so, if it wasn't necessary for them, they wouldn't do it.
- Can be a stim for the child/adult—stims come in all shapes and sizes

Repetitive interaction isn't a mindless activity to your child as you can see from the small list. This form of being doesn't cause your child to become "more autistic" or "stay autistic". I mention these phrases because they are bantered about and you may come across them.

Enabling your child to engage with toys and environments the way they choose to is supporting them and their needs.

When seeking support for your child such as Occupational Therapy or any other kind that you may choose or has been recommended to you, there are some phrases to watch out for that could be red flags of concern.

Phrases such as corrective play and controlled play are two that come to mind. Imagine being a young child with some or all of the aforementioned sensory challenges and an adult sits you down and tells you how to play? Tells you how long you should be engaging in an activity? Stops listening to you and disregards what you need to feel good. How would you feel?

Your child has the right to play the way they want to. They have a right to engage with the world at their pace. The right is theirs to learn about who they are, without being constantly corrected or have the toys or equipment taken from them.

There is plenty of time for your child to step out further into the world and engage in other experiences. They may need longer time spaces in each phase of their development than neurotypical children. They most likely will, because they process everything differently, they will do things and need different ways of learning and experiencing life. The more they are rushed or pushed to do things by someone else's mindset the less likely they are to want to engage with other people.

Unless your child is hurting themselves or others, take a step back to watch and learn about why they are needing to repeat. If you cannot figure out the reason but they are happy, then simply accept and quit worrying.

My son has had many different repetitive needs from toys to puzzles pieces to food types, DVDs, shoes, clothes, people, movements, stims, outings, routes on walks and he still does at almost, 17 years old. BUT most of them are different to when he was 5 years old. Your child will develop and grow just as my son has and their interests will vary, some by a lot, other not so much.

Over the past few years, I have been witnessing many conversations between neurotypical parents and carers and autistic people discussing repetition in various activities. The questions are almost always about how can a parent stop them from repeating activities or asking how they can find ways to reduce the amount of time using a particular game or activity.

The answers are predominately the same, let them repeat as much as they need! (Bear in mind the experts are the autistic adults being asked this question.) They have been young children and teenagers; they usually have gone through the same or similar needs of repetition to your younger children.

Trust that your child knows what they need and be at ease with it. There are countless examples and scenarios of families whose autistic child wants to be on their computer or iPad "all of the time" and how lots of arguments and meltdowns, sometimes destruction of equipment and homes have taken place all based around repetition. Most of those children and young adults begin to self-regulate once the carers have taken a step back and stopped putting boundaries on their usage of a tablet (for example) or swing, whatever it is they need to repeatedly engage with.

At first, the child ups the time spent on their preferred activity, this is usually where the parent can get a bit panicky and step in too soon and think the child is getting worse. If they wait a little longer, maybe a few more weeks, that is when you will see a change. The child begins to realise they do not have to be on it or with it all of the time. They get to relax because they know that an adult isn't going to put a time restriction on the activity, which can create a resistance to stopping because they are unable to fully relax into it.

Many autistic children and adults have little concept of time once engaged with something they enjoy and find solace in. The fear of having someone take it away for a short period of time or maybe even a week, a day and then being forced to find something else to fill that gap is so intense and unpredictable that they increase the use of it.

Once time has gone by where the parent has not given any restrictions or threats of having it removed, they begin to relax. Naturally they find they do not need to be on that activity as much. They know they can have it whenever they are going to need it, this enables them to enjoy other activities.

My son did this with his iPad. Years ago, he wanted to be on it for hours at a time, sometimes 2–3 hours for each session. Whilst this was sometimes challenging for me because I wanted him to hurry up and finish to get on with the rest of the days routines so he didn't get to bed too late (for example) I knew, well I learnt that the more I pushed and tried to rush him the slower he got, sometimes he would need to go back to the beginning of his little iPad routine and start again!

I watched and realised every aspect of his choices and order of apps were important to him. Rushing him or stopping him out of the blue because of my own frustrations seriously messed up his flow. So much was going on in his head, sorting and organising, learning, making sense of. More interestingly, the activity he was currently enjoying was also a stepping stone towards his next choice. If I stopped the iPad routine, I then messed up the rest of his day's activities, the flow would be different, everything out of whack—timings—everything!

I realised that this shook his whole world and would cause him to not only go into a very distressed meltdown but sometimes a shut down too. So exhausted would he become from the overwhelm of thoughts, sensory needs and emotional upheaval that he simply couldn't cope. All because I needed him to get on a bit quicker.

Once I stopped doing that, I saw a change in his behaviour. He began using his iPad less and less, he wasn't panicking and trying to be on it as much as possible in case Mum took it away. He still uses that iPad, it is still positioned in the kitchen, where it has always been. The difference now is he goes on it once a day—he uses only one app rather than the 30ish on there and he is on it for 10 minutes every morning. He did that all by himself.

I have heard many other stories like that from other parents who pulled back from them needing their child to stop the "repetitive" activity to find the same behavioural changes my son had.

It really does work—repetitiveness is extremely important to your child if it is what they do. They are gaining so much goodness from doing the same activities over and over, there is no need to worry. I promise you, unless it is dangerous—it is OK. They will not be stuck in that stance forever. It is a part of their ever-changing development and exploration of the world, their part in it and how they can learn about who they are and how they tick. The most important relationship your child is going to have, is with themselves.

Repetition has a part to play in that learning, particularly when you think about the additional sensory needs they may have. Repetition is logically necessary because of the intensity or underwhelm of any sense that is being experienced for them.

This now takes you nicely to the next chapter which is all about routines and the need for them. There will be some cross over reasons as to why they can be extremely important for your child. Repetitive and routine activities are similar in many ways, as well as having standalone valid benefits…

Chapter 17
Routines: Why Are They Important?

Routines can be a big aspect to an autistic person's daily living. The importance of them is more than just needing to be in control. I have heard this term used many times during my son's life and personally I found it lacking and unjust as a precise assessment.

Whilst I understand how this word has become normalised within language used to describe the autistic children's behaviours, I feel it is a phrase that needs picking apart.

My reasoning behind this is, the phrase "needing to be in control" can sound like a person is being selfish, bossy and obstinate. It can certainly rub other people up the wrong way and I have seen it create a battle of wills between student and teacher or child and parent many times both personally and professionally. It has been a too common phrase said amongst some who work with autistic children and adults as well as it sometimes being quoted in assessments and reports.

The "needing to be in control" statement fits into the same category as "inappropriate, picky eaters and lost in their own world" I feel it is time to highlight the invalidity of such phrases and why. Words are powerful and they do hold quite a steadfast quality to them that can mar your child's relationships with the many people who cross their path.

Once words are a familiar sight, they automatically come validated, they can go on and remain unchallenged for decades. Instead, they are accepted labels and phrases holding an autistic child hostage to a trait that is negative, inaccurate and without further investigating other truthful reasons to how they are behaving and more importantly, why.

If a child is not doing something a teacher or parent has asked them to do and wilfully refuses, rather, needing to stick to their own agenda (routine) it does become a battle of the wills.

This is unhelpful and nobody gets what they need, most of all the autistic child who is being misunderstood because of a constricted mindset.

There are always reasons for behaviours, ALWAYS. It really isn't as black and white as is often made out by the assessments made and the language that is used within it. These kinds of words (amongst many others) are lazy labels and judgements that prevent an autistic child from being understood and their true personalities known.

Within all organisations, there is a language used that you do not use anywhere else. The medical profession has words and phrases that are specific to their work and assessments, as do social services and psychologists to name just a few. Often during a meeting with a combined parent and professional, the parents can be at a loss in some of the language used by the professionals, it just isn't their everyday dialect.

During such assessments and meetings, unfamiliar words and phrases can get easily lost amongst the emotions and tiredness a parent/carer is often feeling. Sometimes the meetings are scheduled in a small-time frame, restricting any longer discussions to filter out anything that needs rewording. Added to that is the huge amount of content that needs to be discussed, these tiny but powerful words and phrases used to describe a child get left unchallenged or fully explained and justified in relation to their behaviours.

The concern then is as they continue with their young life and their support system/network or setting changes—the labels do not—they stick and that child is forever known as "controlling or needing their own way all of the time" as if it is a terrible personality trait that needs stopping.

Routines can be seen as a need to be in control, like I have already stated if seen as a negative it can prevent a support setting from helping a child create a routine for fear that they will not be able to function outside of it and they become fixed into a particular routine FOREVER!

Although in recent years, the understanding of routines and their purpose is becoming more understood, there is still plenty of work that is needed to ensure that all autistic children have their routine needs honoured throughout their whole life.

This chapter will help you see how routines support your child and why they are crucial for their wellbeing. If your child seeks or creates routines, let it be known, they need them.

There are autistic children who do not need the security of a routine or they may need only a few, none of these pages are suggesting that all autistic children do it this way or that. For those who do, I hope this chapter can give you some understanding of the power a routine brings to your child's life so that you can ensure all who cares, also accepts and supports their need for routines and rituals.

There are Teachers, LSAs and other professionals involved with an autistic child's health and education who have a wider understanding as to why routines are important to the individual. When this is the case, it creates a different assessment outcome because the behavioural aspect will look different. Rather than seeing a "rude or stubborn" child they will understand their needs and reasons behind a routine driven life.

However, there are still many who do not, this is mostly due to a lack of correct and adequate training in autism and its many dialects of languages and behavioural needs. The other reasons are usually environment driven, for example a school system may not feel they can provide a child with an individual need for specific routines that do not tally with the schools current "one size fits all regime".

Therefore, it is not the child or even the staff that need to change, more so the whole education system so that it can be inclusive to all children— that means radical changes—maybe it is time for those to happen, after all it's been since the 1880s that the education system became compulsory for all children in the UK. Although it has had tweaks and introduced many ideas of methods of teaching, the concept of its intended outcome is the same, with little thought to the individual needs of an extremely diverse clientele.

Although there are exceptions to this sweeping statement—on the whole, schools are not meeting the needs of neurodiverse children across the country and the world. This isn't about bashing the teachers and support assistants of our lands, definitely not—this is about supporting them to change the system—up date it and create a healthier and non-competitive learning and explorative environment for all children of all neuro types.

Ok, back to routines! All humans enjoy and need routines. Being autistic is not exclusive in this department. We create them for ease and predictability, somehow, they help make our day feel right and comfortable. Just as the chapter on repetition said, routines too can create a flow that eases us from one activity to another all in the safe space of familiarity.

Right from when we are born, we are trained into routines that mostly fit into another person's socially accepted curriculum. (Usually, the parents or carers which is usually because of the need to go to school or work)

Naturally, from birth we eat when hungry and sleep when tired but because our parents have already been trained to eat at specific times and sleep throughout the night the two do not marry up, causing one of the parties to be exhausted…which is usually the parent/carer.

Therefore, we as new-borns are eased into aligning with the rest of the household and by the time, we are pre-schoolers (mostly) we are living with routines in sleeping, eating and many other personal rituals. It's how our whole human existence is set up.

My point is routines are a part of all our lives and we eventually find a comfort and familiarity in having them, even if they were not made by ourselves, rather an exhausted parent when we were babies.

Sometimes we start to get bored by our own created routines, perhaps we have been doing them for years and we do not get any joy from them anymore.

Many routines can send us into autopilot, which can be both a benefit so that we do not have to think too much but the downside can be that we are not connected to life, we do something but are thinking about something else, never present, for the adult locked in a routine—they can become lazy.

Think about the routine of a car journey, something you do day after day. Do you sometimes find yourself not remembering going through a roundabout or a set of traffic lights? Or putting stuff away and then suddenly wondering if you had and having to go and check because you cannot remember doing it?

When boredom sets in, those changes in routines are made and new adventures are created, it feels like a big deal for most of us when we change them, even worse though if someone else changes it for us, or circumstances out of our control happen that make a cosy, familiar routine dismantle. This can feel discomforting, creating some anxiety and frustration until we can re-establish ourselves into some kind of rhythmic pattern.

Autistic children and adults are no different, routines are created very quickly by many, sometimes as quickly as doing a particular thing a certain way only once. Then it becomes a routine that needs to be repeated every time in exactly the same way.

My son navigates his life by having routines and rituals for everything. This crosses into all areas of his current life at home, school and respite. Thankfully for him his teachers are excellent at supporting him, his assessments and reports are worded in a way that tells even a stranger reading them that he understands life through routines, they are a valid and accepted part of his personality. More so they are accepted as a crucial aspect to his wellbeing and understanding of his environments. Everybody gets the best of him when he is held within his familiar patterns and routines. This includes being—outside, indoors, eating, bedtime, order of playing with toys, books, bath and every aspect of his life.

This is so important for him as a developing young man. As he matures into adulthood and eventually lives away from home in supported living his needs will need to be met. The sooner a carer, advocate or professional support can make it clear that routines are a necessary part of an IEP or care plan during the assessment processes the easier it will be for everyone. It will become so in drenched into the needs of the person, you normalise it instead of it being seen as abnormal or a problem to be changed.

Of course, there are times in life when routines cannot be kept to, unexpected changes can happen at any time. When this happens, it can cause a great deal of distress to a person who needs routine for a multitude of reasons. Having b plans and sometimes c plans is something I urge you to consider. This can then become a part of the routine timetable (kind of) also having emergency strategies and alternatives to replace things when disrupted can help stabilise a stressful situation.

This is when a creative imagination and a skill to quickly problem solve is needed! Having an autistic child in your life can help you with this skill, you do learn to be flexible in your thinking and creativity, there is almost always another way to support a child whose routine has fallen apart. Finding another familiar activity or object/toy is the better option whenever you can.

Over the years I have heard phrases such as "You can't make it a yes world for them all the time" or "You can't let them have their own way all of the time" or "If you let them win every time they will never learn".

These are the phrases you need to listen out for and nip them in the bud as soon as possible. There are ways to support compassionately the need for routines and how to fulfil them. The more that happens the easier it will get for the autistic person to cope when sudden unexpected changes do happen. It is inevitable that they will, that's life and even with all the planning and preparing in the world some things simply cannot be avoided. That is when your child will find it difficult and distress will ensue on a major scale.

Why then, would anyone want to or expect a person who needs routines to cope with that kind of change on a regular basis? Why should they? It can be trauma inducing long term and create a major mistrust of new situations and people. The more you take away from a young autistic child because it is seen as "inappropriate, obsessive or stubborn" (I use these phrases as examples of what language is bantered about to justify removing routines) the higher chances there are of them retreating and having an unwillingness to try new experiences. They remain anxious, unhappy and disorientated, not being able to relax and enjoy their life.

If routines are needed, taking them away can feel like being in no man's land, a feeling of standing without a floor, lost in a space not knowing where to go and how to anchor down to feel safe.

Earlier on in this book I have spoken of trust. The need to create trust in relationships whomever they are with is crucial to enabling an autistic child to develop and be interested in new experiences. If they are consistently pushed or stretched too soon, what actually happens is they retreat and become smaller. A feeling of fear of life and its unpredictability builds because all of the coping strategies within a routine that they have cleverly created is taken away.

This isn't a nice way to live life, distress increases which creates all kinds of physical and mental problems. It is an unnecessary strategy, especially when it is totally possible to help and support an autistic child within routines they need whilst still fully engaging in life.

Everything is a stepping stone to something else. The theme through this book is to nurture the child and their needs even if at first you do not understand why they need to do what they do. The more support and time taken at this young stage will determine their lives and the thriving of it in their future selves.

I know and understand this because my son lives his life by creating routines for himself in everything he does, as do many other autistic people all over the world. Guess what? They haven't remained in the same bubbles of routines and rituals, instead they have become confident and thrived, gaining independence in many aspects of their lives as they are able to cope with.

New routines are constantly created both through their own doing and those that were unavoidable (unexpected changes) The point is no one has become "stuck" in the imaginary place that is often assumed by others with their advice on how to prevent routines from becoming too, well routine like!

This is through no malice of theirs, rather a lack in understanding in the meaning and importance of routines to the individual and how, instead of stopping—enable the routines so that trust creates a quieter and calmer state of mind which can develop whilst the child learns about themselves, their sensory sensitivities and environments.

Telling the Time

Routines are a valid tool for telling the time for many autistic children. My son has found and created numerous methods to help him communicate his needs and navigate his way around the day which aids his independence. Many he has created by himself for himself and I have been the avid learner and he the teacher. Passing on his wisdom and examples feels right as I have seen the positivity his routines have provided him with in all of his relationships and experiences.

Some autistic children will grasp the concept and will readily tell the time of day by a clock. However, there are many who will not, no matter how much you would wish them to. There can be numerous reasons for this, which will differ from person to person. Some examples are:

- They have dyscalculia (number dyslexia); this can make remembering concepts of numbers and what they stand for difficult or impossible to remember. Looking at numbers, particularly within a small space close together such as on a clock can make it very difficult to see them clearly and at the same time figure out what the time is.

- Time telling is too demanding—to final—creating a stark "end" feeling within them that they find extremely upsetting.
- The concept of time gets lost and simply has no real meaning in relation to their inner compass of existence—meaning they live totally in the now (all of us when babies and young toddlers automatically have this skill, we eat and sleep when we need to, as opposed to when we are timetabled to); eventually, we are weaned away from our natural functioning rhythms and routines are created that fit into everyone else's patterns and societal expectations and rules, work, etc.
- For the sensitive sensory overwhelmed autistic child, they are so connected to the environments, their physical (sensory) experience is so intense that time (human concept) is harder to grasp and adapt to.

Routines created throughout a day can replace the clock telling time method. Each activity that happens is a stepping stone towards the next one. Therefore, if one aspect of that step is removed or interrupted then the whole day, or some part of it is disrupted which can be what causes major upsets and meltdowns. It's like someone coming along and removing an hour or two from the clock. One minute it is, say 1pm; the very next, it is suddenly 5pm. This would cause most people to feel very odd indeed in a multitude of ways.

A feeling of incompleteness, like being left hanging in the air with nowhere to go, no anchor to secure you into the next stage. For children who have vestibular sensory or executive functioning, even interoception and proprioception issues having a routine disrupted can be catastrophic for that person. If you understand or know about those four senses, you will know what I mean by that.

Each activity becomes a section; a block of time used within the chosen activity, this can be anything from eating a snack or having a drink, to a full-blown meal, a look at a book or a longer activity of iPad or swimming (for example).

This is why when a new activity or experience is offered, even if it is seen as a pleasurable one. For the person who needs the routine to help understand the order of the day, or even what day it is, the new activity can be extremely upsetting. (It may not be because they do not want to do the activity or that they wouldn't enjoy it.) Timing is everything, and this is a skill that you will learn on how to negotiate new experiences.

It is like having to squeeze in another activity into a short time restraint. For example, it might be 4.15pm and you have a task that will take you 45 minutes to do. Suddenly someone comes along and says you have to do an additional task but still be finished by 5pm. You have to renegotiate those 45 minutes which can be difficult, discomforting and stressful. It will have a huge knock-on effect for the rest of that day, upsetting everything—which for many it is annoying, for the autistic routine needing (relying) on them, it can be confusing and very tiring.

Another demand that can deeply affect a person who needs and thrives within a routine day is hurrying them along. Say, for example you are running late for something and you need to leave the house for a specific time. Telling them to hurry up can create a problem; this is for the same reasons as adding a new activity and having to squeeze it in, hurrying up a person means they have to speed up their activities which can mess everything else up for the whole day.

Missing out parts of their routine (which is what would be required if you wanted them to hurry up) can be impossible for them to do, it leaves everything unfinished, incomplete.

For some autistic children and adults, this is major, full-on distress that can last for hours. When my son was younger, he would be extremely upset if this did happen on the few occasions it did, he was inconsolable for hours. I would end up being late anyway because he needed comforting and time to calm down, It was counterproductive and I quickly realised he just couldn't cope with this interruption of events.

So, as much as I could I would avoid doing this, although sometimes in life this isn't always possible, with careful pre planning on my part it has mostly become a thing of the past.

It is important to add that as he grew (just as with the other examples I have shared) he has developed a very clever coping strategy, one that I am not sure I could do myself.

If on a rare occasion we have to hurry up, he will still need to play out the activity, whatever it happens to be. So, he will close his eyes and go through the activity in his mind on fast forward. It is incredibly clever and a major coping strategy that enables him to be able to move on without upset.

Obviously, he prefers to complete the task physically but if there is no choice, he can go to this (fast moving strategy) and complete his activity. He has done this when on his iPad, looking at books, playing with his soundboards. Of course, he needs space and time to be able to go through the activity in his mind this way. Therefore, it is vital that I tell his other carers this is what he does whenever he needs too. He will not be able to just stop one activity and move to the next. Giving him the time to go through it his way still takes a few minutes.

Another point to make is he cannot always do that, some things are just to set in stone, the depth is too deep. He will simply close his eyes and stop, shut down. Once the person asking him to hurry or stop eases off, he can then resume the activity.

Another aspect of this same strategy is if we go out and something has to change. Sometimes we cannot go to a particular field that we use on one of our walks because the cows are in there and the gate is closed and locked. So, he will stand still and close his eyes and walk that part of the walk in his mind on fast forward, then happily turn around and continue our walk back. Another example is when we go on this walk, we often meet a friend who walks with us, then leaves us at a certain point to return home. If on the odd occasion they cannot join us, he will still stop at the point they usually leave us and go through the motions of saying goodbye and hugs. He doesn't mime it out physically but he waits and closes his eyes to do it in his mind. I think that is an excellent skill to have created for himself.

The challenge was for me to recognise what he was doing to give him that tiny bit of time to complete the tasks in his mind. It is definitely a lot quicker than what the actual activity would usually take, so these days when we need to hurry up most of the time we can. I was so thrilled when I clicked and realised what he was doing, I observed him enough to figure it out.

As I have already mentioned, sometimes, although rare, this is not something he can do, instead he will stop in his tracks. Things like walking faster he cannot do. Each step has a meaning, the timing and feeling of it is intense and crucial. If I ask him to hurry up, he freezes, I know him well enough to know this is his way of saying I cannot do that, I just can't. This can be tricky when crossing a road, but if I try and hurry him, he just stops, nothing will move him, which creates more waiting time for any passing traffic and at the same time creates more stress and possible accidents. Instead, I have become a good traffic controller. (There are other reasons he walks very slowly, mostly to do with audio and other sensory sensitivities)

This may seem (to some) unreasonable on his part; I do not see it that way because I know him and have learnt to understand his limitations. I have seen that when he can he will develop a new strategy that can help him move along more quickly. If he doesn't, it means he cannot. I have learnt to accept that and so help him out by ensuring he is safe. Now he is almost17, I feel he can tell me when he is stuck and cannot cope with a change, this example of walking quicker is one of those times.

If a person had a physical disability that prevented them from being able to walk (for example), we wouldn't expect them to suddenly get up out of the wheel chair and start running because we needed then to move more quickly. It is the same principle for my son in this instance.

When he was younger and was inexperienced in himself as well as a lack of life experiences to help him develop strategies for himself—any changes in a routine would cause him inconsolable anguish. He was too young in every way to be able to cope with such changes, he was like a blanket being thrown about in a washing machine, never really knowing which way was up or what any of it meant. In the example of walking faster, he used to lay down in the road, whatever the weather, mud, puddles anything. He was so consumed with intense sensory challenges that he did not understand and so his routines, familiar toys and patterns helped give him a small amount of clarity and peace.

As he grew and developed, he began to create coping strategies of his own. He no longer lays on the ground, so at least he is upright and can be seen. In other instances, is the use of photos and picture symbols to help him express himself. I would also give him photos of what could come next so he didn't have to try and scramble about in his brain and try to figure out what it all meant, which—created that feeling of free falling and fear of the unknown.

He now has AAC devices (a working progress) as well as his social board with real photos of places, people and order of events, to this day, this is still his favourite method of seeing his routine and what is expected to happen whether at school, home or respite.

For the most part though our go to strategy was, and still is to enable him to have his rituals and routines (sometimes it means I have to negotiate time scales to cater for these) then as each year goes by, he matures, his trust builds, his life experiences increase and he naturally develops his own coping skills and flexibilities.

At 17, he still needs routines and rituals for every part of his day but because he has had a combination of trust in the adults around him and he is learning to adapt at a pace, his pace (without thrusting him into a constantly changing environment on someone else's terms.) He can feel confident in being flexible and able to cope with small, even bigger changes or unforeseen disruptions. He has learnt that the adults in his life always have his back, they respect him and his needs, doing the best they can to support and guide him.

Here are some examples of what he uses with a set out order of routine of individual tasks during a particular activity:

- When eating food—he will lay it out in a certain order, eating each piece in the same way every mealtime, he will get the foods out of the fridge in the same order too.
- When out in the woods or any familiar country walk, he will use the same route every time, including going to the same trees or landmarks in order (as he has gotten older, he can deviate a little bit from that as long as he can reclaim the original pathways to continue.
- When interacting with his sound books, he goes to each one and presses the buttons of each book in the same order every time.
- He watches the same DVDs each day of the week in the same

order.

- He gets dressed in the same order each time.
- Puts on his shoes using the same number of times to get his Velcro shoe fastened
- Brushes his teeth in the same way every time
- Puts his creams on and in the same order
- Touches certain items at specific times within a bed time routine or in between one activity to the next
- He finds things being moved around a room or space difficult (impossible) if it is moved in front of him. Everything has its place—he finds stability and comfort in this

These are just a few examples to give you an idea of what can be required as routine and ritual.

Routines and learning communication and language skills

Yes, having routines can help a non-speaking (in particular, but also a speaking child) learn language and communication. If the carers around the child, pick up on the pointers that the child is giving them.

Firstly, learning what words means can be compartmentalised depending on the activity or part of the routine the child is in. Usually there are specific groups of words used in particular situations. An autistic child can have very clever ways of finding their way around this very confusing and loud world. Breaking situations down into categories (small routines/rituals) can make life that little bit easier to navigate.

I could write a whole book or at least a few chapters on language and communication alone. By that, I mean a multi-language/communication approach. When spending time with autistic children, you quickly become aware that spoken language is only one way to communicate effectively.

I learnt that one of the benefits my son has gained from developing so many rituals and routines is he can understand words spoken to him in a specific context.

Language and socialising can be one of the most difficult experiences for an autistic person, whether they use spoken language or not. Neurotypical people use so many nuances such as sarcasm, joking, abbreviated words and phrases, tones that mean different things, some even use words that do not match their intentions, to name just a few. It is almost like a secret coded language (or at least that is how it can seem) which can leave an autistic person feeling confused and completely out of the loop.

Therefore, for the young autistic child just starting out, using smaller routines to learn spoken language and what it means, makes it easier to remember. It breaks down sentences, phrases, words, contexts, tones, sounds and word—action—meaning for the child to be able to store it in their memory, a kind of brain zip file.

For example, my son knows and understands thousands of words, yet if a word is used that he already knows and understands in one circumstance but is then used in a completely different one, he will find it difficult to understand what is being asked of him.

Here is a more specific example, he uses a spoon to get some hot chocolate onto a plate for an activity he enjoys every day for years and when I ask him to get the spoon, he understands and gets a spoon. However, when we started baking at home, I asked him to get me a spoon assuming he would understand—he didn't. He did his best to fathom what I was asking him for he knew he had heard the word spoon before, but he had no experience of using that word within this experience.

That is just one example, he does it in every situation which I am now aware of, so can show him in any particular situation what I mean.

This can happen with places too; a child may know where a toilet is in one café or restaurant or know how to use the cutlery but in a different setting it can be completely unknown. Every place and situation are brand new; everything is different so it's like starting from scratch again.

By having sectioned routines with different activities and places, the autistic brain can very cleverly organise those words and phrases into categories so it makes it easier to find. Even when those words are the same ones in a multitude of situations, which of course they will be. To the person needing to use this strategy it isn't seen that way. Each place and experience are unique and therefore different, completely different.

Once you learn and understand this as their carer/support or advocate you can make sure others know this so that your child can go through their day with more understanding and confidence.

As I have previously touched on, routines can help the child know what is coming next. It paints a nice clear picture or pattern for them to follow, so if writing happens now (for example) I know that swimming (for example) happens next. This is why social boards and first and then photos can be really helpful. This helps them to know what is expected of them. The compartmentalisation of their day keeps everything easier to understand.

An autistic brain is an extremely busy one, the sensory perceptions and pathways are unique and complex. With your newfound knowledge of the senses set out in previous chapters, you can now see just how much information their brains are constantly processing.

Another example can be: a child may know how to take off their shoes and put them on independently and competently in a specific activity. You offer them a different setting for a new activity which requires them to take off their shoes, you may see that they freeze or look to not understand what you are asking them. New place, new activity, yet same language, except to them it isn't the same because everything else is different, so the words you speak will feel and sound different too.

Obviously, this can vary from child to child and some autistic children will not have this challenge. It happens enough for me to include it in this chapter to hopefully help avoid major misunderstandings. Knowing it as a possibility means you have a better chance of recognising it if it does happen so that you quickly adapt.

You may by now have figured out that routines can create a feeling of safety for the child who needs them. I do not mean in the sense of getting hurt or having their life threatened in any way that is obvious to an outsider looking in. I mean the safety wellbeing of the child who is already feeling extremely anxious because the world is confusing. Senses are processing on a higher scale than most humans can comprehend. This in itself can give the feeling of anxiety and confusion which can lead to a fear of an environment and experience. The routines that become familiar with the language compartmentalised, rules laid out clearly, time frames understood, then becomes a feeling of safety.

With all those familiarities from the routine day, you will see a calmer, happier child. You will see their true selves shine, their personalities reveal themselves, rather than a constantly scared and stressed-out child who is unable to engage with anyone or anything because they are unable to settle into a comfortable and familiar space.

None of us are at our best when we are highly scared or stressed out. Personalities change dramatically for anyone who is under huge pressure. Have a think about when you have been highly stressed, scared even, worried, overwhelmed, exhausted, confused. Are you happy, coherent, willing to engage in meaningful conversation and interactions with others?

Add onto that maybe a headache, extremely thirsty or hungry, maybe your backaches, added on maybe you have lost your phone or your car keys, oh and you now feel extremely nauseous.

If you felt all of those things and you were in an unfamiliar setting or activity, you didn't understand the language being spoken to you because you are disorientated, even though each individual word you have heard before. Can you see how disabling that would be for you? Although this might seem a little over the top. I can assure you for many autistic children and adults this is not an exaggeration. Routines can create a living experience that gives calm and meaning to their day. Please, honour children, or indeed an adult who you may know at a work place, college or as a friend—their routines are there for valid and important reasons.

Decompression is another thing that routines can help with. We all need down time, relaxation space. We all have our own ways of chilling out.

A familiar routine can give that much needed space to let go of all pressures, sounds, smells, visuals (whatever it happens to be that creates sensory overloads for the individual)

Routines created by the child can and will give them the space to relax. They will not have to try and figure out what is going on, deal with unexpected sensory inputs, language, demands and uncertainty. Instead of being stretched and pressured by painful anxiety and fear they can unravel, decompress and finally relax. A bit like what a massage or a meditation, a glass of wine, chatting with friends, exercising or whatever your hobby is, may do for you.

Like I said at the beginning of this chapter routines can make us lazy if we do not challenge ourselves or become too entrenched in the same thing day after day but equally they can help our day flow along real nice. Only the individual can decide this for themselves, which is what I am highlighting here with this chapter.

If someone came along and said you had to change your schedule because they felt you had been doing the same thing for too long, without a choice but to adjust, without warning or any comprehension of your needs and reasons, how would you feel about that?

If routines give autistic people any of the benefits and possible resources that I have suggested here, you can see how removing them can now be seen as cruel, unjust and counterproductive to that person.

Working with the child and helping them to create routines in any area of their daily life, can help you have a positive relationship with them. You will learn so much about who they are and how they tick. You will see their personalities shine. The feeling that you cannot connect with your child would disappear, rather than believing that they may be locked in another world that you cannot enter, you will know they are doing their best to engage and thrive in the world we all live in.

The difference is, they need specific methods and tools to be able to do so as life gets easier for them it also gets easier for you. I mean that you will find parenting and supporting easier, because you have allowed yourself to learn from the child/adult you are living or working with.

There is much you can and will teach your child, but you too are a student. The child is the teacher, still, today autism and sensory sensitivity is misunderstood, the only people who know about this stuff are the autistic people of this world. Let them show you who they are, without the need to change and fix every aspect of their existence.

Once you step into that vibe, many of your worries will disappear or at least a huge amount of them will. Have more trust in your child and their autism. The world is big enough for them to be in it just as they are. Of course, there will be aspects they will need and want you to help with, you have plenty to organise, support and teach. However, when their behaviours are unharmful in any real way because there isn't any danger to their health or wellbeing instead, enable their behaviours to unfold as you observe so that you can learn all of their languages; physical, mental, behavioural and sensorial—you will see just how much they are communicating and why.

NB: Words typed in brackets are phrases and labels I have heard used by others and are not words I personally use or accept as legitimate in relation to the chapter's subject.

Chapter 18
Stimming and Ticks

Stimming and tics can be a part of an autistic person throughout their whole life. That said, anyone can stim in various ways, for an enormous number of reasons. This is all completely individual; it is highly unlikely that the same two people will stim for the same reason or emotional reaction. As with the rest of this book, I am talking about stimming and tics solely in relation to autistic children and adults.

Tics are like a "sneeze type behaviour"—quick, fast and usually involuntary—this has its own spectrum which vary to one-off sounds and movements to a diagnosis (or undiagnosed) of Tourette's Syndrome.

Tics can occur at any time for many reasons, for some people, tics can occur when they feel more relaxed, yet whilst they are focused on a task the tics can stop. There are people who tic, but when they sing, they stop (just one example) for other people, their tics happen whether they are busy doing something or not.

Stims are generally more patterned, rhythmic and as a fluid response, interaction (communication) or reaction to an experience felt by the person stimming.

They can be connected to the sensory input a person is experiencing at any one time, although not always. If a person is having a sensory overload or a particular sense is deeply felt with an activity or experience, they are having—stims can increase in speed and intensity.

For example, when my son is near waves he will stim with his hands and arms in a familiar way every time, they are big arm and hand stims that can be super-fast, he is so joyful that he expresses this with his laughter and the intensity of the experience enables him to overflow and filter through his stim. In this instance, for him—he is both expressing his joy and having a conversation with the ocean as it creates waves and sounds, he responds (like in any conversation between two people) with his physical and vocal stims.

There is a lot of research out there to delve into to get a more in-depth knowledge of stimming and tics on specialised websites and social media autistic led groups.

My son has a vast array of stimming techniques and tics in his vocabulary that changes as he develops and experiences the world in its multitude of ways. I will give you some examples to help you gain a clearer picture of the variations.

Sometimes his tics are short term, lasting only a couple of day or weeks, whilst others have been with him for years. Some leave for a while and return at a later date. Some are noises and sensations coming from different parts of his body, (such as clicking knuckles and finger joints) others are physical tics and stims. Over the years of watching, listening and learning I have naturally learnt what a tic and stim is, for him.

It is all a part of his complex language, that is what I have learnt from him. This form of his expression helps me to communicate with him, you see his tics and stims help me understand his feelings. He interacts with the environment on every level (physically, emotionally, intellectually and sensorially) in an intense, intimate, intricate and beautiful way.

Sometimes it is his tics in particular that develop when he is having a physical developmental surge, like a growth spurt.

I recall when he was beginning some hormonal and physical changes around the age of 12, he began making some throaty sounds, like small sharp sounds, gruff like…he then began touching his throat area a lot. At first, I thought he had a sore throat, once he was checked out to eradicate that possibility, after some observing and asking, we realised he was feeling his Adams apple beginning to develop. He could feel the change in his throat and it felt intense. His voice was beginning to drop as he was entering the next phase of puberty.

Actually, as I am writing this, he has entered a new phase of his puberty development, he is almost 17 and his Adams apple is continuing to grow. For the men reading, you will be familiar with this feeling, as a girl I have no idea about Adam's apple and their growth feelings. I cannot recall my brothers mentioning it to my parents when they were going through it. My son is very physical in his awareness of stimulus, he feels everything so deeply and his Adams apple is quite big and prominent which is why he is making throaty sounds again. Maybe that is the difference between him and my brothers, his sensitivity enables him to feel his body growing way more than they did.

Within this particular phase of his maturing and development, he is adjusting to the change, experimenting with it. He is trying to understand it and adjust with it by creating different sounds that are short and frequent. He isn't distressed about it, more fascinated, he is showing an awareness and acknowledgement and is interested and accepting of it.

Here is a list of some other tics he has had over the years of his life so far. This can give you a few examples of what a tic can look like, obviously there are endless types that any human can have in an array of ways. See this as an introduction and invitation to the language of tics, to enhance your awareness of them.

- Throat tics—sounds of various tones, octaves, volume and length—short cough sounds but not an actual cough
- Nose tics—sounds or snorts or sniffs
- Eye tics—blinks or closing eyes and opens quickly, moving eyes from side to side
- Hand tics—short finger flicks
- Finger, knuckle and toe clicks
- Mouth tics—pursing lips together and making a pop sound—opening and closing his mouth fast making a raspberry sound
- He can add sound to all of the above—often added with a giggle
- Sharp, quick movement with his head and neck, arms and body with a sound added with it

Stimming is a huge part of his existence and interaction with his environments, they are an expression of him and his feelings as well as his communication with the elements, energy and other sensory internal and external stimuli.

Some stimming examples of his are:

- Hand flapping really fast and sound added which can be both loud and soft
- Hand clapping (especially when eating anything, wherever he is)
- Large body movements like a leap into mid-air and a vocal sound at the same time
- Lip sucking and eyes blinking at the same time—sometimes hands and arms flapping at the same time
- Laughing—yes laughing can be a stim too (obviously laughing is also an emotional response to something he has enjoyed) it is also a stim for him. He can laugh and laugh for hours sometimes, he loves the feeling it gives him and he can literally do it for hours, it

is stunning, and highly infectious!

- Spinning around when he was younger—he did this a lot, he never got dizzy, he doesn't do this one anymore
- Spinning objects, anything he could get to spin he would (only very occasionally he will do this, these days.)
- Stim with objects in his hand—flapping them in front of his eyes very close up particularly when younger, he does still do this but very rarely
- Opening and closing doors, sliding doors especially, open close, open close, open close, blinking and flapping at the same time
- Lights on and off on and off on and off, blinking and lip slapping at the same time
- Banging on side boards of the kitchen, doors and windows

I will remind you that the above lists are only a few examples of tics and stims, that are unique to him, he has hundreds of others, too many to list.

There are thousands upon thousands that others use in a variety of ways and for even more reasons. I am certain that my son has many more that I have not picked up on or recognise as a stim or a tic. I have an awareness that I am continuously learning about him and his many communications and expressions with the environments and experiences he is in and interacting with.

Throughout his life we have never suggested that he stop any of his tics or stims. It genuinely never crossed my mind to do so. Sometimes his stimming is loud and constant, lasting for hours at a time. Even then, did we never tell him to stop. If they became too loud for me to cope with for any reason, I would remove myself from the space he was in. I am extremely audio sensitive so sometimes I would need to go to a different space as I would become overwhelmed by the loudness of his stimming, putting on headphones to decrease the input into my own ears. This also helps a lot too when I get a bit stressed, I need to move, so I will dance or sway whilst wearing headphones so we both get what we need without upsetting each other.

I have already mentioned his beautiful relationship with the water element, since he was a baby. Watching him stim when in and around water is really an amazing thing to witness.

Especially when at the ocean with the waves crashing onto the shoreline, he stands and as they rise up before they crash onto the sand, he will be there like he is orchestrating the water, I have some incredible camera shots of him doing this. He stims with music, food, mountains, animals, people and most visual things, especially when they are new experiences. Like I have said *stimming is a huge part of his personality and demeanour. It is how he expresses himself in response to and as a as a form of communication with everything.*

Stimming can increase and decrease, fluctuating constantly depending on a person's wellbeing. If they are feeling unwell, poorly or ill, they may need to stim more or less than their usual amount. The feelings and sensation that arise with any type of illness, even a gentle cold can create intense feelings that need a stim to help process them and help them flow through the body. The stims may change slightly or they may develop new ones, unique to the particular feeling say, a specific kind of physical experience gives.

Stimming can increase if a person is tired or excited about something. Or they may be extra stressed or had a difficult day, perhaps at school something happened that was extremely challenging for them and so the stimming heightens as a way to help filter through the intensity of whatever it is they feeling. It could be because they are sad or angry about what has happened.

If a person is told to not stim or is reprimanded for doing so, (this happens a lot in school settings) then once out of that environment they might need to stim intensely for quite a while. Some forms of stimming may not have anything to do with the current environment or situation—more so with a memory of an experience that happened that day. It isn't unusual for a child (for example) to come out of school and go into full-blown stimming mode once in the car or home. A place they feel safe and free enough to let out all the supressed emotions they masked that day.

It's a bit like someone having a really crappy day at work, maybe an argument with a colleague or a deal didn't happen—and once home they cry or rant to a partner to help make sense of the situation, problem solve or to just let it out and express it.

Sometimes, memories can come up that happened years, months or weeks ago that will be so real and clear, as if they are experiencing it at that very moment—stimming may happen whilst they are reliving that memory, because the feelings they felt at that time are easily accessible to them through the memory of it. All humans do this, I am sure you will be able to recount a few experiences, good and not so good that stirs up old feelings of crying, laughter or even anger when you recall and tell someone about it. Although temporary, they are just as real as they were when the event happened for the first time.

Stimming and tics, can be repetitive, sometimes all day long, no matter where the person is in public or what is going on around them. Usually stimming will happen regardless of social rules and expectations. For example, if at a cinema, stimming will not stop because they are in a public place where people want you to be quiet and still. In school, stimming may be needed which can be disruptive for the other students but a necessity for your child or adult, where ever they are—at work, school, doctors, library, concert, anywhere.

If a child starts to be reprimanded for stimming enough times, they may stop and internalise the need to do so. Also there are some autistic people that cannot stop and will not respond to being told to stop. This does not mean they are being rude; it simply means they cannot stop because the input of the information they are experiencing requires a reaction, usually a physical one so that they can literally keep functioning and staying upright—many adults have, unfortunately learnt that stimming can create huge problems for them. This can result from being bullied as a young child into adult life. Or from disappointment and lack of understanding of the necessity and purpose of the stimming (for the individual) from carers and teachers. All that can contribute to them being shamed by their behaviours.

For some people, stimming increases when there is a lot going on, whether that be visually, auditory, physically, emotional or because the sensory information they are receiving and have access to is massive. Overloads of the senses in a number of areas can mean the stimming can be more intense and become louder, faster and last for longer periods of time.

Historically, such behaviours were forcibly stopped, without knowing the reasons why. Ignorance was rife with regards to autistic people and all their behaviours, especially stimming It was seen as "too out there", too obvious (needing to be hidden), too strange and an unacceptable behaviour for society to cope with. Silent hands was a strategy that was (in some places it is still enforced) used to stop a person from flapping or moving their arms and hands. This was a method of repeatedly telling the person to put their hands on the arms of a chair and keep them still. Sometimes they were told to sit on their hands, worse still some had their arms and hands strapped down!

Back in the day, self-expression, especially in public, in any emotional way for all humans was seen as common, lowbrow, embarrassing, even unacceptable. As we have evolved, we have become more openly self-expressive, not only physically but emotionally too.

There is still a way to go in allowing ourselves to let go of embarrassments in expressing ourselves of a genuine feeling of delight or despair. My feeling is when all humans get comfortable with themselves in how they feel and are able to express it without fear of ridicule will they be able to accept the stimming behaviours of others. (We can see through our cultures today in 2022 we are focusing on being seen as individuals, it's important to all of us to be seen and heard as we are, unique and of value.)

Stimming is an emotional and physical response/reaction to something else. Throughout this book and its chapters on the different sensory processing experiences one can feel, it is not surprising that stimming is needed to help filter through the exterior and interior sensations that are felt by the individual.

Have a think about your own physical reactions to some extreme situations or stimulus. Maybe a really loud bang or other sound that comes out of the blue will create an involuntary physical or vocal response? Some of us will scream when an unexpected sound or scare occurs. Some of us jump or run, duck down or put fingers in our ears.

Some sounds or experiences can make a person hum or sing things like, "lalalalalalala" sometimes a thrilling experience say at a music festival or concert will drive one to scream, shout out, dance, jump, sway, cry…close their eyes and smile…all of these things are really like stims in the way that they are a reaction, conversation or response to an external/internal or both sensation or feeling one is having.

Feeling anxious or scared, excited or happy can create physical movements in a person in forms of perhaps, tapping a pen on a table, constantly tapping a foot or leg, flicking a pen on and off, drumming on their body or moving around because the feeling of nervousness or excitement is too much to hold in the body.

An anxious or excited expectant parent has needed to move around whilst waiting for the birth of their child. Waiting for exam or test results, I have seen many a person create some amazing stimming type behaviours.

It soothes us, it helps the feelings of intensity, good or not so good flow through our bodies. Without the stim-like outlet, we somehow feel overwhelmed and feelings of panic can well up. Or we can feel like we will explode or implode, like a pressure bubbling up until the release comes, resulting in the body automatically moving as well as making sounds to assist with the intensity of feeling which helps us filter it through, making room for the next feeling we have.

For the neurotypical human who has no sensory processing challenges, doesn't have Tourette syndrome or any tics, stimming—like behaviours are still a part of life. It is a human response to something happening around them or to them. An expression of joy, sadness or even terror, fear or enormous sensory input too much to cope with by simply standing still. The body needs to move or create another sound to help filter it through our bodily system. It's basically, expression to put it simply.

Is dancing a stim? Can it be classified as such, I would say yes, dancing is a great huge stim that most humans find irresistible to do when they hear, feel music that they like.

There is a lot of "stuff" on dance stimming online, in relation to autistic people as well as discussions and research into dancing in general and whether it classifies as stimming.

I am a great lover of dancing, I do it every day of my life in one form or another. I dance for different reasons, sometimes I just need to move my body without music, simply to the rhythm of myself, sometimes it is to relieve myself of tension, other times it is to music that I particularly enjoy. I have many different types of dancing and some of my moves wouldn't be regarded as dancing rather what is seen or considered as stimming. Sometimes my dancing (moving my body) is to meditate—so for me, dancing is a form of stimming, it is in a communication to sounds of some form or another—it enables me to feel the vibrations flow through the body and it feels fantastic.

Stimming really isn't that weird at all, it is a very clever and useful tool the body uses to help with the flow of strong emotion running through us and back out to the world, like a form of communication, a conversation with the environment via our bodies.

Why do autistic people stim? Maybe now you have read through the previous chapters on all the senses you will have some idea on how to answer that question. In this chapter, I delve deeper into the world of stimming in particular to help introduce you to some of the reasons, and types as well as giving suggestions on how to help a stim be safer for the individual if they are causing harm to themselves or others.

It is different for every individual as to why and how they stim. I couldn't possibly answer for anyone else, I can, however speak for myself and give you examples of how and why my son stims as well as share with you what other autistic people have told me about their stimming. What I do know is that if a person stims, it is because it is a necessary part of their life. If it wasn't, they simply wouldn't do it.

Some stims are used as a distraction from other events or experiences, such as noise, visual or from an interaction or demand that is unpleasant for the person. Others are used as a kind of filter system, a dulling down of intensity that can reverberate through the body's various sensory systems. This can be for sensations that are both unpleasant and pleasant.

Some stimming types can be harmful—such as hard banging on the head or face. I mentioned way back in my earlier chapters that my son used to head bang the walls, windows and floors every day for hours it was very stressful to witness. It was worrying as he was a baby as young as 14 months old which he did right up until he was around 2—3 years old.

I remember placing cushions where he was so he could have a softer surface to head bang onto. I would use myself as shield for him whenever I could which wasn't always possible. He had a large bruise and sometimes gash on his forehead for a few years. I spent many sleepless nights worrying that he would end up with a serious brain injury or not wake up at all, due to severe ongoing concussion.

Back then I was inexperienced with these behaviours and what they meant for my son, I did not know what to do to help him or why he was needing to do it. We got him checked out to see if he had earaches, headaches, or any other kind of physical pain, there was nothing. He continued to do it daily, sometimes he would hit his head so hard, it was difficult to bear. He would never cry as he did it, did he feel any pain I will never know if he had pain or not, maybe the sensation of the head banging was less than the discomfort he was feeling that made him do it in the first place. Kind of like a counter balance, distraction or release.

I knew he had a reason and that he was doing it when he felt distressed, I just couldn't figure out what was causing it.

I have spoken of this previously but will explain in more detail as it reiterates the possibilities of finding a less harmful stim if it is causing physical damage.

One day I held him tight, like a squeeze really, I held his head and body tight to me under a blanket, rocking. He suddenly became relaxed and stopped needing to headbang. I did this more and more, eventually being able to ask him if he needed a squeeze. He started to approach me voluntarily and make a sound that I made to him when asking if he needed a squeeze. I don't know how to write the word that would describe the sound I made, but it was a sound he could mimic which meant squeeze.

This was a major breakthrough, he needed the squeeze and it had to be tight, sometimes he wanted it just around his head sometimes his whole body.

This was a stim that was potentially harmful to him, bruising around his forehead and a constant swelling was definitely cause for concern, so I needed to help him find another way to soothe whatever it was that was causing him to headbang so frequently.

He was very young then and everything was new and incredibly overwhelming to him, especially sound, he had not yet learnt how to self-regulate the incoming audio that was bombarding his intensely sensitive ears. Somehow the squeezing of his head and body helped release the tension and energy build up in his ears and head, I gave him a space he could let go of it somehow. To this day, very occasionally he needs a squeeze—sometimes just around his head—its acts like a pressure valve letting out excess build up. As I have already explained he regulates himself and the incoming sounds by physically using his outer ear lobes like volume control dials, I have seen many autistic people use this strategy with their audiology sensitivity.

If a stim is causing harm to them or others, finding a different way to alleviate the discomfort is very important. If the dangerous stim is stopped one way or the other, the need to release will still be there. It is vital that you help the person find an alternative stim to help filter out what causes the original harmful stim in the first place.

The issue with not finding a replacement outlet and investigating why the need for that particular stim exists means a more /harmful stim may take its place. The other possibility is that the pressure, discomfort, distress, or joyful feeling of emotions or feelings they are experiencing that created the stim will be internalised. This, to the outsider may look like a problem is solved and all is well. For the person experiencing the surges of sensations, though is a very different story.

Internalising the need to stim is incredibly difficult and exhausting, it can create more problems for the person than the stimming itself (even when the stim is harmful to them personally). Remember the need to stim is a strong response or reaction to something, therefore stopping it from happening will have a strong impact on that person in many ways.

Anxiety and frustration can build up, and new self-harming ways can manifest. This can usually lead to personal self-harming such as scratching, banging, hitting, biting, hair pulling, skin pinching/ pulling/ scraping, face slapping, nail biting and so many more.

If a person creates enough anxiety build up and sensory internal pressures where there is no outlet or self-expression release, the body can shut down. It almost has no choice; nobody can carry that amount of internal tension and emotional build up forever. It can also create illness such as headaches, nausea, tummy upset either diarrhoea or constipation to name a few. A person who is stopped from stimming will become more anxious, seriously, even severely so.

A sadness of not being understood and accepted will build where the person will feel isolated and lonely. The feeling can be like you have been put into a strait jacket, caged and unable to express yourself freely. This may sound over the top, please believe me, this isn't an exaggerated explanation.

Shut downs can last for days, some last for a few minutes or a couple of hours. Many an autistic adult who has masked their need to stim or tic because (for example) they are in a work place where it isn't acceptable has resulted in 3–5 days, sometimes longer shutdowns. This has meant they cannot eat, sleep properly or talk to anyone. They shut themselves away and usually isolate until they are regulated again. This is extremely distressing for the person experiencing this. Long term this can be seriously damaging to their health in many ways. There are many links and social media groups where autistic adults can further educate others on such matters.

I thought it might be useful to give some more examples of different stims that I have heard about over the years, some are my own, as well as my son's along with other autistic people I have met in the last 17 years:

- Hair pulling, twirling, stroking, manipulating somehow
- Finger/knuckle/nail biting
- Skin cutting, biting, pulling, pinching, scratching, banging, stroking
- Using specific material like, soft fury fabric or shiny sequin type pillows, cushions, toys, materials (there are loads of those type of materials available, my son loves to stroke sequin blankets and we have a few around the house)
- Sensory toys and objects such as squeeze balls and toys, stretchy toys, objects that twist and change shape, like Rubik cube style toys
- Particular music and songs
- Particular TV shows
- Particular blankets and fabrics, including clothing
- Using specific vocal sounds of their own (including screaming or using particular words, repeatedly) talking or singing/humming

- Doing specific movements using various parts of their bodies
- Rocking
- Swaying
- Running
- Jumping
- Leaping
- Spinning
- Climbing
- Stamping
- clapping
- Drawing, painting using fingers, hands, brushes or any other equipment
- Water activity, for example could be running a tap, swirling water, splashing water, drinking, spraying
- Pressing buttons on specific objects for the sound or colour they create over and over again
- Running specific objects across their skin or face, lips
- Being squeezed
- Eating specific foods, textures, drinks, ice
- Blowing bubbles
- Spitting
- blinking

Remember this is a broad list, each one I have mentioned can be presented in a variety of ways. Such as, for example: running may need to be in a certain place at a particular pace, wearing no shoes or using different levels of pressure, say stamping, stomping, sliding, hopping or super-fast. There are so many more that other autistic individuals will tell you of, including your own child or client.

Some stims will be used for both exhilarating experiences and feelings as well as unpleasant ones. Not all stimming is because a person is distressed or overwhelmed by something. They can be because the feeling is so wonderful the need to express this through the body somehow is a celebration of that experience.

To be clear I mean that a particular stim, let's say (for example),—jumping can be used in the same way (visually) for both happy feel-good sensations as well as equally (in intensity) unpleasant painful sensations. The intensity of the feeling or experience is the same but for different reasons and so the outlet expression will be the same, even down to the noise. (Remember, the story of my son laughing whilst being jumped on, when he was actually scared and in pain?) Although this example is not of a stim, it shows that what may look to an outsider watching the person stimming is a happy experience, it could in fact be very unpleasant and vice versa.

This is also because whilst the stim is happening there are other sensory experiences and pathways at work running simultaneously. Remember the interoception sense? Which can confuse happy and sad expressions as well as—not being able to regulate crying or laughing or use it to match the emotion being felt.

Both nonspeaking and speaking autistic children and adults use stimming to express their experience, whether that is joy or not and anything in between. It is so much more than a physical act. Language comes in many ways and stimming is a valid and purposeful form of communication. Just as dance, singing, miming, drawing, storytelling or signing is.

The key is to figure out why the stim is there, particularly if it is dangerous or harmful, because, as previously explained, knowing why will help you help find a safer, yet just as satisfying replacement.

Some stims are needed when performing bodily functions, such as eating and drinking. This may mean that sitting down and eating in the conventional way is not possible. Stimming may be required to help that person process and deal with the sensory sensations of the food and its flavours, textures and feeling of swallowing and digesting. Eating is an intense sensory experience for all of us, for extra sensitive autistic children and adults this is tenfold.

This is possible for toileting and bathing—stimming may need to happen whilst the sensations of the bodily function are happening. There is always a reason an autistic child does something in a particular way. The stims around toileting may be because of the internal sensations, the noise, the place, the whole thing it could be to help dilute the intensity of the feeling of toileting.

Some children need to stim when they are listening to others talking to them—for example if an autistic person is rocking and finger or hand flapping, closing their eyes and blinking to name a few, do not be offended by this or presume they are not listening to you. This is a way of being able to hear and process what you are saying. Remember stimming happens for feeling the vast spectrum of emotions any person can feel.

A few examples of food and toileting stims that my son likes to do are: He likes/needs to eat his dinner standing up, most of the time. He likes to use his fingers and as he eats, he has tic's that are unique to his eating routine. He also stims using his food as well as his body. He uses his voice when he is chewing food so is quite a loud eater, clapping at the same time. He isn't making chewing sounds or slurping sounds; this is an actual throat sound to help with the auditory sounds that happen when eating. He will often sway or rock, leap across the kitchen and bang on the kitchen surfaces and cupboards. He will put his hands to his ears and rub them after he has swallowed each mouthful.

All of this enables him to eat with more ease and most importantly, pleasure. I see it as none of my business how he chooses to eat and why. He needs to eat and if he finds the stimming helps create a more pleasurable feeling whilst he does, I am OK with that. It is clear that, for him eating is an intense sensory experience that affects him deeply, including physically. The auditory sensors are hypersensitive and the very act of eating creates a strong pain/sensation and discomfort for him.

Toileting for him has similar stims, he needs to close and blink his eyes, he makes different sounds with his mouth and throat at the same time as well as holding his ears, it's a massively intense experience for him.

Proprioception sensory needs are also a possible reason a person may need to stim. The need to release or feel pressure within their bodies. Some stims, depending on what they are can be of great support for the proprioceptors within our internal body system, as already mentioned in the proprioception chapter.

I hope now stimming can be seen and understood as an integral and valid part of the autistic child/adults being. Getting comfortable around someone who stims is really the best support you can give. Rather than finding ways to stop it (unless it is seriously and genuinely harmful) accept it, let it be and spend time learning about why they do and imagine how it feels to that person.

The more you learn about it the easier it is to accept and the less strange or uncomfortable it feels to the observer.

Generally, in life most humans spend way too much of their time worrying about what others are thinking about their behaviours. Trying to fit in and not be ridiculed or judged for wearing certain clothes, speaking in a particular accent are just a couple of examples, the truth is it can be any kind of difference.

This is an opportunity to begin to help yourself become less of a worrier about what others think. Typically, an autistic child will be who they are wherever they go, and quite right too. They will not worry about other people staring unless they are made aware of their behaviours in a negative way.

Although humans can be judgemental when faced with a new experience that we do not understand, or that veers away from social "norms or acceptability" we can also be extremely accepting, kind and compassionate. The more autistic children are supported in all of their needs and expressions, the easier and quicker others will accept and stop judging or teasing stimming behaviours.

We all need to be free to express ourselves and whilst some of us find it difficult to do so, most of us wish we could be braver, more confident in saying what we mean or doing what we want when we want. Dancing to a favourite song in a supermarket, why not? We worry people will stare, I say give it a try have a little sway or dance and get used to being seen as different—this will help build your confidence and it will definitely also support your autistic child or client when in public and their need to stim.

Who cares who's looking!

Chapter 19
Executive Functioning
How It Relates to the Sensory System

Although Executive Functioning isn't a part of our sensory system per se, it can be affected in a multitude of ways for all neurotypes, especially for the autistic, sensitive person.

Therefore, I felt I needed to include a chapter on how it can be directly affected in one or more of its aspects in relation to over or under responsive senses.

There are eight areas of the Executive Functioning System that make up the cognitive behaviours of all human beings:

- Flexible thinking—how we adjust to unexpected events or quick, out of the blue changes—the ability to figure out how to readjust
- Working memory—How to keep a tab on where we are throughout an activity or experience without getting muddled or forgetting where we are or what comes next.
- Self-awareness—how we see ourselves in its entirety and how we are affecting others or being seen by others, as well as how we are being affected by others (so boundaries can be tricky to establish or notice).
- Planning and prioritising—how can we set and meet goals, whether they are from ourselves or from others instruction. How

do we manage this?

- Task initiation—getting started on anything at all—getting out of bed or writing a letter (for example) or even to begin to move from one activity to another. (transitions)
- Organisation—how do we organise ourselves to function each day, such as getting dressed, brushing teeth or getting on a bus at the correct time.
- Impulse control—can we control this easily or do we just go ahead with an action without first checking if it is safe to do so, or affecting another person?
- Emotional control—can we monitor our own emotions? Can we recognise what we are feeling in relation to something or someone else?

As you can see from this list, it covers a lot of our human functions. Each bullet point indicates in brief, how we survive and its impact on being able to navigate our way through life and all of its many decisions making demands, whether they are positive or negative, decisions are always having to be made, choices decided…

Having Executive Functioning (EF) issues is another stand-alone condition, you do not have to be autistic or have sensory processing challenges to have EF difficulties. Yet having sensory sensitivities can affect your executive functioning in a very big way.

If you have already read the previous chapters on the other senses, you can probably start to build an understanding of how some or all aspects of EF can be affected.

Throughout life, most humans will have some struggles with their EF for a multitude of reasons. Sometimes when we are feeling poorly, extremely tired, grieving, in shock, angry, scared, confused or in a panic.

For some people, being hungry can affect some of their EF skills quite dramatically. Usually, our ability to concentrate on a task or keep our memory bright and functioning are the main functions that are affected if we feel or experience any of the above.

Once you understand what EF is and have an understanding of the sensory challenges an autistic child may have, it is easy to see that what may look like an intellectual disability is in fact an EF aspect that is affected. I want to be clear, sometimes there is an ID (intellectual disability) at play also, I only make this point because it is usual (not every time) for a child or adult who is being assessed for autism to get a diagnosis for intellectual disability as well.

Whilst this may be true in some cases, for others it isn't, rather the EF capabilities are compromised. Some may say that this does qualify to be seen as an ID, others will not.

What I have learnt is that once certain areas of difficulty have been realised, such as an EF issue, different strategies and wording can be used that will enable the person to understand what is being asked of them, like following instructions for a task (for example) and their "intelligence" is no longer in question.

This is why it is crucial to get under the microscope during assessments, gathering as much information about a (child/adult) in order to fully support them so that they do not have to be wrongly labelled with something for the rest of their lives.

When different teaching methods are used and alternative ways of supporting them are applied, the child or adult can begin to live more independently in a multitude of ways. They will most definitely feel respected and less treated like they are lacking in intelligence (a broad spectrum covers what intelligence is anyways). That, too, is a huge stand-alone subject—what is intelligence?

For example: Let's look at the Task Initiation aspect of EF. If there is a difficulty there, one solution and supporting tool are the use of social boards. They can be tailor made to fit with exactly what it is the person needs those visual prompts and reminders for.

Of course, as with most assessments during a child's very early life, some areas will be unpresentable at the time of initial assessment processes. There may be times when a child is deemed intellectually disabled because they are not yet mature enough in their mental, emotional or physical development for an assessor to correctly spot any difficulties there.

This is why some assessments are put off until a child is around 3–5 years old. There are many assessments that can be carried out with a baby right through to adulthood. The key is to be very specific about what is being assessed, which areas of the child's development are being looked at and why.

Assessments can be made fun without the child knowing they are being watched and marked on how they interact, respond or play. Having separate sensory assessments carried out and at numerous stages in a child life can ensure that nothing is missed, whilst at the same time the child is being seen in a realistic—real time line.

This is the ideal preference, (although not always possible currently due to a lack of resources) to be able to carry out the continuous assessments on a more regular basis. However, with the knowledge you have gained from reading this book, learning about the benefits of observations and additional research into the sensory systems you are tooled up (so to speak) enough to be able to monitor a child's progress in all sensory related areas as well as their executive functioning ones.

As I have said in my earlier chapters, you, the main carer is the key, the constant person in the child's life who can keep their progresses and challenges up to date. We know children do not stay the same throughout their whole life. There is a developmental process that happens however small or big that is as well as knowing they ebb and flow for all manner of reasons.

Sometimes we do not easily notice how a child is developing if we do not continue to observe them, along with offering new opportunities their way.

The danger of labels such as "intellectual disability" isn't necessarily the label itself, rather what another person does with that label. Sometimes a child can be held permanently to a label that is attached to a formal diagnosis.

Although a label is NOT a diagnosis, it is often seen as one so is set in stone that the child is A, B or C. (whatever the label is) Therefore new experiences and activities are not considered because the diagnosis report includes labels that are considered to be fixed, unchangeable or seen as incurable. Of course, any assessment can be updated, so be sure to keep an eye on that so that the child's progress is kept up to date and amended wherever necessary.

Executive Functioning (EF) is one of those areas that can be completely misunderstood and therefore undiagnosed or recognised as an issue. Instead, other labels are put in its place such as Intellectual Disability (ID) or Global Developmental Delay (GDD) amongst others. Ensuring it gets included in any assessment report is key to fully understanding the child's neurotype. By having EF looked into as an official assessment means details are logged, so that an exact support plan can be created for the child as early as possible.

Let's look at each of the eight aspects of EF and see how it can relate to our sensory system, we can then see how that sensory issue will affect aspects of the EF system in practical terms.

Flexible Thinking

Flexible thinking is the ability to find another strategy or a different way of doing something that is unplanned, an out of the blue happening. A sudden change of plans or something breaks, like a toy or a cup, perhaps a planned outing is disrupted because the place is unexpectantly closed. (This has happened to us a few times throughout my son's life and it cause a great deal of distress) This can be an extremely difficult thing for many autistic sensitive children and adults to cope with. Switching to an alternative activity, a plan B, even with photos and incentives of finding something the child really loves to do can be unsuccessful. Switching from one idea to another an impossible task.

We know that all of the senses can be both over and under responsive, we also now understand that they are all consuming—being able to then cope with an unexpected change or happening without warning can bring up all kinds of other challenges in the EF areas.

I will use a fire alarm as one example, Schools, Nurseries/ Kindergartens/ Preschools and workplaces will usually have scheduled fire drill practises. Whilst some preparation can be made, occasionally they are not, in order to help staff and children can get a sense of what happens in a real-life emergency situation.

If a child has an over responsive auditory sense, the sound of the alarm will be excruciating and therefore terrifying. This will immediately disable them into being able to think clearly about what they need to do to follow emergency instructions that arise out of the blue.

Whereas if planned and prepared, perhaps the child can be given ear defenders to block out or dampen down the extreme intensity of the fire alarm. They will then show that their EF skill in regard to flexible thinking (an out of the blue interference in their current activity) are more capable than when they were in a trauma state because of their over responsive sensitive ears.

If the child/adult has an under responsive auditory sense, they may not respond to the sound of the alarm at all. They may not hear it, or recognise it as a sound that means a fire alarm. They will not be able to understand why everyone is suddenly moving around quickly and getting into lines ready to evacuate the building. The lack of auditory input can create confusion and affect their EF—ability to think quickly and reorganise themselves accordingly.

If the child has a vestibular sensory issue and the fire alarm goes off— the sudden movement of all the people in the room at once can create an overwhelming sense of giddiness and disorientation. This will directly affect their ability to think on their feet and figure out what is going on and what they need to do and why, even when they have been told many times and experienced a fire drill before.

An interoception sensory issue can affect the ability to sense danger from inside our bodies or from external dangers such as with this example, a fire threat. Therefore, the child or adult may show a lack of urgency in relation to the situation in hand. If, however the child has an over responsive interoception sense, they may get extremely freaked out at the sound of the alarm even though they have been told it is a practice. They may not listen to the instructions or may have a really hard time concentrating on what is being said because their sensory system has gone into overdrive panic. Therefore, their EF skills of being able to think clearly and safely will disappear.

You can see from just these few examples of other sensory challenges how the EF of a child/adult will be compromised, whilst if they were not experiencing such sensitivities, they would have more able flexible thinking abilities.

Understanding the child's sensory functions intimately and intricately will enable the carer, parents, therapist to fully support and prepare a child for almost anything. In the example of the fire alarm scenario, it may mean that showing more compassion and patience for the child is all that can be done. Or maybe a weighted blanket or their soothing toy, maybe headphones as previously mentioned, will be that something which can soothe them a little during the fire drill. This can make all the difference to them finding the anchor point they need to help them think more clearly.

Whilst in other sensory areas it could mean that visual boards are displayed so that the child can see right there in real time what to do and how to do it. Support workers and LSAs can have a mini visual folder on a key ring or small floppy folder that is carried with them wherever they go or an AAC device can be used.

Knowledge is power, we hear that saying all the time and it is true. The more we know the more we can be prepared for anything as much as possible.

Working Memory

When our senses are overwhelming us, it isn't a surprise that our memories may be affected. Remembering how to do a task that perhaps is done every day can become an enigma. It is as if the activity has never been done before, this can also be due to the flexible thinking aspect of EF.

I know personally when I am overwhelmed with one of my sensory issues, I am unable to remember the simplest of tasks, I usually get caught in a loop of whirring words and instructions without being able to come to any conclusions. Sometimes the only way for me to remember something is to back track to a point in time that re-triggers my memory of that particular task.

This has happened during the creating of this book, I can lose my train of thought if I either have any background noise or I look up too often. My thoughts cannot go any further until I have eliminated the other sensory inputs.

Over the years I have been told about this by numerous autistic people of all ages. Many folks who live independently will create lists for themselves so that they can remember what to do either at home, work or school.

When a person's EF is affected in this area, visual lists are extremely important, they can be the difference to having a successful day or a day full of disharmony and stress. Visual and other reminders can create a day without confusion or disappointing someone else, like a boss or work colleague because they have forgotten to do an element of their job that they do every day because there wasn't a visual timetable or list of chores. With all the other distractions such as constant conversations, demands, sounds and unexpected events, memory recall can very easily be distorted and interrupted, completely scrambled to the point of a complete freeze in actions and thoughts.

Visual social boards for children and adults are brilliant. They can be put onto iPad and phones as well as being a board up on a wall in all the rooms of the house or classroom areas. Having a notepad with some bullet point instructions of what order to do a set of tasks so that none are forgotten can be a lifesaver. These days there are watches that can plan your whole day, which can be a very helpful tool for anyone who has EF issues.

If the person is feeling poorly or stressed, tired or hungry to name but a few reasons, the memory can be affected and once again difficulties can ensue if a visual board or list of instructions is not in place.

This is often an area of difficulty that no amount of practise will improve it. Of course, I am not saying this is the case for every person or situation, sometimes the memory recall will strengthen for certain tasks if done often enough. I am highlighting that when EF difficulties are present in a person, it is not to be presumed that practise and repetition ensure that memory is improved – lists and prompts may always be needed.

My son needs visual boards in every aspect of his life. He created for himself a visual board made up of mostly real-life photos. He can use some symbols now he is much older but when younger and with limited life experiences he needed real life photos. I say he created it because when he was very young, about 2 years old he did not understand what symbols of a playground were or what a symbol of a banana was. He was so young and inexperienced in himself and the world around him he could not fathom what a drawing of something was.

He showed me he needed something different to help him understand. When I took a photo of the park and a banana, he immediately understood what they meant, because it was actual real-to-real images. Now he is older he can understand many symbols, you see he has vast experiences as well as built up cognitive skills and learning all kinds of symbols in school and home having learnt what their meanings are.

A symbol of a tree or a playground (for example) was not real to him, it had no context when he was very young. He could figure stuff out if it was the real photo of a tree or a photo of the playground we were going to. Makes sense really, a literal thinker (as I am too) means just that, literal. Therefore, symbols of objects, people, places and foods can be meaningless to a child with no life experiences to give context or comparisons to or for someone who is a literal thinker, or both!

The symbols and pictures used for sign language and social boards can be learnt (like any other language) in time, my point here is when a child is very young using real actual photos can make their understanding much easier and less stressful.

He also began using items such as particular shoes or boots, jackets and trousers that he had previously worn for a particular outing or activity. This helped not only to know what was coming next but also aided his memory recall. This method has continued to be a favourite of his as he has grown and matured. Although he is now beginning to retain memories of tasks and in what order more frequently, I believe this is because of all the other support systems that are in place for him which for most people are invisible as we now have a finely tuned set of tools and cues that he uses on a daily basis.

Most of that is incorporated in the routine element of his toolbox! The existence of a routine-based life has enabled him to learn memory recall at his own pace. Throughout his life he has continued to skip forward with some tasks without needing to use the board. We still use the board as a back-up because there can always be something that upsets him in some way and disables (momentarily) his ability to remember tasks. So, the visual board is there to help him get back on track. A bit like a notebook or an instructions manual.

For many adults, writing a list on a board, their phone, or on bits of paper is enough. For tasks such as getting ready for work in the mornings, from getting out of bed to brushing teeth, washing, dressing and eating breakfast. The lists can be specifically detailed or like a bullet point system which can be something that may needed for the whole of their life.

Writing lists is something we all do from time to time, I used to try and keep tasks in my head, not realising I could write stuff down. I think I thought it made me look stupid if I needed to do that so I didn't bother. Or maybe it just didn't occur to me that I could do that. Wow, the difference it made writing things down, the stress you do not even realise you are put under by constantly trying to remember everything in your head.

It leaves the mind free for other things, instead of filling it with constant noise of voices telling you not to forget this and that, then ultimately forgetting many things because it is just too difficult to remember a whole day's tasks! Especially when other sensory issues and challenges are constantly at play on top of having to socialise and communicate with other people.

Life doesn't have to be so difficult; it isn't a test to see how much you can do without help, making life as easy and comfortable for ourselves is surely the kinder and more loving way to be. It also helps to get tasks done way more efficiently and quickly, probably the most important point is it can make an experience fun.

The brain cannot function when the body and senses are under pressure, it stands to reason that all aspects of executive functioning is going to be affected and compromised in one way or another.

Self-Monitoring and Self-Awareness

This is an interesting one because when we are all new born we do not have a sense of self in relation to others or our environments. This typically does not manifest until around the age of two years old, sometimes a bit sooner or later. The sense of I and me in relation to who or what is happening around us kicks in.

This can be lacking or highly acute creating feelings of paranoia and constant anxiety and worry of being watched. It can almost feel like you are under a bright spotlight and everything you feel, think, speak and do is judged by others, when this is over responsive.

When under responsive, you can easily carry on with your day without showing an awareness of what other people are doing. You can appear self-centred or uncaring of other people's needs and feelings. This extends to the self too so not being aware of, for example wiping your mouth after eating or having an awareness of nudity or needing to be discreet if having a wild wee!

My son still has difficulties in this area, if he needs a wee when we are out in the rural countryside where we live, he will continue to go through the motions regardless of who may be about. This is a constant learning and he always needs reminders that he needs to hide behind a tree or a bush!

Being accused of being selfish or inconsiderate can be commonplace for an autistic adult particularly if the people around them do not know of their challenges, or do not understand or accept them.

Helping a child to become aware of others feelings can be another lifelong exercise. Not always, it depends on many things, usually consistency of being around specific people can help but not completely eliminate the difficulties on seeing other people's perspectives and needs. Humans are by nature inconsistent, even fickle and do not always say what they mean or mean what they say so trying to figure out another's emotions or needs can be a minefield of challenges.

It is much easier if a person is completely direct in what they need and what they feel and why. This can be one of the most common differences between autistic and neurotypical people.

This can be misunderstood as an inability to show compassion to another person. Feeling compassion and empathy and not knowing how to show it are two very different things. This can often be the case for autistic people, expressing their compassion is the part that can be difficult.

The feeling of compassion or empathy can, in fact be intense and all consuming. Sometimes though there is a complete lack of understanding in why a person (usually neurotypical) would feel a certain way about something, so being compassionate will be difficult.

Learning to be self-aware is something that can be taught as a skill; however, it is another of those areas that may need continuous support in day-to-day life.

Using mirrors are a great way of helping a person see themselves in action and relate the words you use when acknowledging them. Such as saying their name in front of a mirror or using facial expressions to show what a happy face or sad face looks like.

Being patient is key, using the mirror activity may not be something a child wants to do, looking at themselves can be overwhelming for a multitude of reasons. It might be something that can be slowly and naturally built up as they grow and develop to help them grasp the self-identity and self-awareness concept.

I had mirrors put up in our house that were low down so that my son could see himself naturally, when he was ready, he would walk up close to the mirror and pull faces, open and close his eyes and practise smiling. He does this more as he has grown—to this day he will spend time looking in the mirror smiling or pulling different facial expressions. Snap chat has helped him with this skill too as this makes it easier for him to look at himself on a screen because he is filtered out by the different apps and images they create. He can see it is him in the picture, yet it is less confronting than say a mirror or camera.

Planning and Prioritising

As with the Memory aspect of EF this is an area that will benefit greatly by using visual boards and pictures. Writing lists in order of importance can be the key to a child or adult having an easier day in work, school and home.

School can be a very tricky place for an autistic child for so many reasons I could write a whole book on that one subject, although I am sure having read this book you can see how difficult a school day can be for them.

In relation to the school day's planning and prioritising, major misunderstandings can happen on a daily basis if this is an area of a student's needs that has not been either recognised by the parents or the teachers as well as the student themselves. Often the child will not know how to find a solution to the problem that they are getting into trouble for on a daily basis.

This can include things like, not completing homework or forgetting PE kits or other items for the school day. Completing assignments or following rules and criteria can be extremely difficult for a person who is struggling with EF issues.

If you think about Executive Functioning and all of its functions, School life fits into all of those categories of potential struggles. The day is full of having to remember tasks, equipment, how to get from one class to another (particularly in High School), organising homework schedules and so on.

This can affect students remembering to take PE kits home, phones, homework even coats. This can cause serious frustrations and financial struggles for parents if they are having to re buy specific parts of a school kit.

If an autistic person you know is having consistent trouble in this area, it is highly likely they have executive functioning difficulties. This becomes more apparent when the person is into high school age, as it is then they are expected to be self-sufficient. They will need help in pointing out the issues and finding solutions that can assist their being able to prioritise and pre plan for jobs and equipment that needs to be taken into and out of school on specific days.

Part of this area of difficulty is that school is school and home is home, combining the two is something that doesn't compute within the reasoning department of cognitive thinking. This is why it affects homework completion for many students, over and over again. Constant detentions or other school punishments will make very little if no difference at all, it will however create a low self-esteem issue, they will feel anxious and become depressed, knowing they are disappointing both teachers and carers but not being able to find a solution on their own can be soul destroying.

The sooner this area of difficulty is realised the better, so that easy strategies which will be unique to the individual can be created to help make their lives (especially in school) less stressful.

Task Initiation

This is another of those aspects that can be misunderstood for behaviours such as laziness or an unwillingness to join in or try new things. From the observer's view point without knowing this is an issue where children can be seen as shy or not interested in many activities and experiences.

Generally, for a person without EF issues in this area, getting started on a task is done without too much thought. Unless of course it IS something we DO NOT want to do such as getting up early in the morning on a cold, winters day might take a bit more task initiation gumption! Or clearing out the garage which has needed doing for a few years…sometimes we need motivation and a little extra determination to getting started on something, even when we know it needs to be done.

What we are talking about here is something different to that. Remember this aspect of our cognitive thinking is strong and needs to be stimulated a lot to get it to either calm down or strengthen. Each day whatever age you are there are many tasks that require initiation.

It starts as soon as we wake from sleep, getting out of bed, getting dressed to eating breakfast, brushing our teeth and all the tidying up and putting away, as well as leaving the house to continue with the next set of tasks.

Everything we do is a task, our lives are made up of constant individual activities, once the EF aspects are broken down it is easier to understand the difficulties that can occur in daily life.

When a young child does not want to join in or "do" any of the activities that others are doing, it can be worrying. Often, unless assessed by the right professional this can be missed as an EF issue. Like I said earlier it can flag up other labels, such as Intellectual Disability or Global Development Delay among others. Neurotypical children generally (not all) will flow from one task to another without thinking, they just do what they do in the moment, sometimes it is getting them to stop which is the hard part!

Like all the sensory functions mentioned in this book there is no straight line, EF too will manifest itself in many differing ways. Some people will need lots of support in moving from one activity to another whilst for others it may be for specific activities or times of the day (for example) this can increase or decrease as the child grows into adulthood.

It is not uncommon for autistic adults to find moving from one place to another very difficult for a multitude of reasons. One example I heard was knowing they are tired and need to go to bed but unable to switch off the TV and transition to the bedroom. It takes so much effort to do this, the stop—start of each activity is a constant separate unit which become so singular that finding a flow between them can be difficult.

Here is a list of some examples of tasks that can be difficult to initiate without support for a young child, as well as a teenager upwards. This is a small list comparable to the vastness of life activities we all have each and every day. However, this list can help you see what is meant by task initiation:

- Getting out of bed each morning without prompting
- Moving from one room to another, however familiar it is
- Picking up a spoon or fork to eat, or just to begin to eat any meal
- Getting dressed—each item of clothing may need prompts
- Getting out of the car to go to another location (even if it is a daily or familiar one)
- Opening a sweet wrapping / any type of wrapping
- Putting down an iPad/phone or coming off a computer or TV
- Picking up a pencil or pen to write or draw
- Stopping any activity once started and starting a new one
- Moving from one place to another—including buildings or classrooms
- Opening a book
- Moving from sitting down to running around in a park (for example)
- Engaging in any new play activity even if the child loves to play

with it
- Brushing teeth, washing, drying themselves after a bath
- Starting to eat or drink

This list can go on, the point is that each step of an activity needs to be broken down so that it is easier to understand why a child may look like they have frozen or have big issues with moving forward.

Sometimes through repetition and support many aspects of task initiation difficulties can disappear as routines are established and kept to. This is another reason why routines can be vital to an autistic person's life (not always) but definitely a valid tool that can help a person have a flow into transitions and activities that somehow assist them to keep going.

Whilst some humans like the stop/start of each individual activity, others do not. It's like the stopping bit shuts down an aspect of their functioning and so takes a big start up and energy to get it going again. It makes sense then that routines which create a constant flow between each step are necessary—movement is then like a continuous melody, flowing beautifully along in harmony. Add to the routines, visual cues and the child may find tasks easier to start and finish.

Repetition can also aid this aspect of EF in young children, slowly building up experience and internal recognitions for them that enable them to start each task more easily. Although even with constant repetition this may still be a challenge.

Support can be given to help the child begin each task without difficulty or missing out on any activities that they want to take part with, such as:

- Visual boards
- Routine

- Repetition
- Singing
- Dancing
- Silly walking (fun)
- Prompting
- Accepting (this may be a lifelong difficulty so not losing patience is necessary)
- Finding a favourite, preferred toy that they can have with them at all times, wherever they are (my son has a lion teddy who goes everywhere with him, if he needs it, this has helped him move around massively). Even a song that can help the child stop and start activities without stress or fear
- Giving some time for the child to gather themselves to begin a new activity (more patience)
- Positivity—not making a big deal about it, instead helping them accept their individuality and not seeing it as a problem
- Egg timers or visual timers (although this can create more anxiety)
- Some children and adults need an item with them in their hand or bag that helps them move from one activity to another enabling them to stop and start on a constant basis. The object (which can be something as simple as a plastic fork, or a piece of fabric, for example) can be the one thing that aids their ability to move from one place or activity to another. This object may seem random or unimportant to others, if this is the case let it be.
- Avoiding using bribes or taking away a favourite toy or using threats or emotional blackmail to getting them to move from one place or activity to another. This will create a deeper resistance to moving, it is often the favourite object (teddy or cup for example) that will help get them to move with time and patience.
- Find a "bridge" item that will help them with the transition part of getting from a to b (this may be a photo of where it is they are going next to carry with them)

As a child gets older some aspects of this may lessen, some may not, so tools and prompts may always be needed to help make life easier at home and at work.

Creating support systems for children means they can use these confidently throughout their lives, this enables them to become more independent in the smallest of tasks, which can create a positive sense of self and confidence. Many aspects of EF can be supported without having to declare all of their challenges to anyone they meet. Unless of course the individual chooses to share them with colleagues or friends. This is especially important when the person begins high school. Some young people get embarrassed about having to have lists and prompts or an aid worker to support them throughout the school day, finding ways that can assist them without the whole class knowing (if this is something they struggle with) is crucial to them maintaining their privacy. High School can be tough for everyone, this is maxed up if the student has some challenges that can be an easy target for bullying.

The list above can help with many aspects of being autistic, having sensory and EF challenges, whilst many will not make any difference. It is a constant discovery throughout a person's life.

When something does work for them, it is worth sharing with everyone who will interact with your child (with their permission and using discrepancy), remember this will become a part of your child's language, an interpretation of their personality and needs. So, the whole of the child can be supported positively, eventually then the support systems put in place become natural, instead of being a highlighted problem or what can feel like a big ask of everyone.

Organisation

When children are very young, this can be missed as a difficulty because usually the child is too young to be able to organise their daily activities, the adult takes care of all their needs in this department. It is only when the child gets older and expectation of self-organisation are expected that this can be seen as a difficulty.

So, like previously mentioned, School can be a place that is affected the most in a young person's life. Every part of a school day is about planning and organising; it can be a living nightmare for the person that is expected to be organised with books, pens, homework, PE kits and everything else that comes with school life.

What may seem like an easy enough planning exercise can become a world of anxiety and overwhelm. Lesson timetables can be very overwhelming when seen as a whole on a piece of paper or on a screen. So much so that every aspect of planning goes out of the window completely, causing bigger problems for the student for forgetting some school kit or a piece of homework (for example)

Like with the task initiation aspect, visual boards or individual reminders and lists can be really helpful for school life.

A diary that can break down each lesson on a particular day including what kit is required which can be helpful. Finding a way to create a bridge between home and school is sometimes the biggest challenge. Throughout my career as an early year's provider most children whatever their neurotype would prefer to keep nursery or school there and home stuff at home. Crossing over the two can be difficult, it's like two completely different worlds that need to be kept separate.

For the autistic person, this can be tenfold. Why would I do school work at home? It makes no sense at all…surely that is why we go to school? This is a logic that many young people have and I totally get it.

Finding a solution to this separation of the two places can be the key to settling into creating strategies to be able to plan and organise for a school day on a Sunday night at home (for example).

Sometimes it comes down to not expecting the child to complete homework, or perhaps, keeping a PE kit at school at all times until it needs washing or having two kits so that one is never forgotten. There is always a way to make things easier if the school and parents are willing to have flexible thinking and be accepting of the child's difficulties. School can be challenging enough without adding to extra demands that the student has genuine problems with.

Planning events into adult life can be as tricky as when they were a child. Using the same strategies such as visual boards, diaries, accepting that different settings can create a gap that two worlds do not meet can positively support the autistic person however old they are.

Work is work, school is school, home is home…and so on, which can actually be a really healthy way to live life for all of us, often we overload ourselves with so much information and tasks that overlap the separate aspects of our lives. Keeping them in their individual boxes can help keep our stress levels down.

Impulse Control

This can also tie in with awareness of self and others. As young children we generally do what we feel right there and then, having no concept of time or appropriateness to environment or other people's needs, especially personal space and boundaries.

As we grow and develop, we are trained by the adults around us to think before we act on something, for a multitude of reasons. Some of which are to help keep us safe, and teach us about personal boundaries, of our own and that of others, all helpful and beneficial.

An obvious example is when we are toddlers, we see a toy we want and so we simply take it without asking first. We do not yet have the awareness to consider the consequences of that action. The need to have it is the focus and drive, when the other child cries or fights back we are completely surprised and confused as to why. Until it happens to us in return, we slowly develop self-awareness and that of others as well as the need and ability to control our impulses.

This is where patience is required with a huge dollop of compassionate understanding of how difficult this concept is to grasp.

Some impulses will be a danger to a child, like the need to touch a flickering flame (for example) or touch a steaming tap of hot water because the steam looks so pretty, repetition of those activities is needed, rather than the avoidance of them. Obviously close supervision is required at all times.

My son was and still is, very attracted to fire or flame whether that is a candle or an actual fire at home or an outside fire. His impulses were intense—so I decided to have an activity that incorporated flame in a safe and fun environment.

The best thing I came up with was a cake with birthday size candles on it, just a few. He was very young when I started this, he would help me put the candles onto the cake, I would light them one by one and with me closely watching he would put his finger near the candle, this would be with my hand on his to guide him but giving him the opportunity to feel the heat, this became a daily activity for a few years. He now understands heat and the need to stay away from flames. I will continue to ensure anyone who cares for Jeorge understands this is still an area he needs close supervision, even with his stronger awareness of danger around fire and flame.

The practising has, though enhanced his awareness of the possible dangers if he does touch flame. Rather than keep him away with a lot of intense fearful avoidance, we have together managed to help him understand and enquire which has eased his need to touch.

Sometimes, however, avoidance is the safest decision, my point is that if there is a safe way to enjoy an activity so that learning can grow, slowly a bit at a time, do it, as it can add to the child's self-awareness and give them time in a safe space to feed their sensory need, whilst learning impulse control.

Executive functioning requires mostly seeking strategies for the person to function more easily in their everyday life.

Here is a short summary of some of the help that can be put into place:

- Create visual boards—start off with a then and now when the child is young, keep it simple and build up to a more complex board as their awareness grows and they show you they are able to follow it easily.
- Use real photos of places, people, building, food etc., when you can, especially when the child is young, then you can start to include universal symbols so the child can begin to read/recognise them in their daily lives as they become adults.
- Keep instructions to tasks short and to the point, no more than 1 instruction to begin with, let confidence build, then add another.
- If the person can read write the instructions and put on the wall, keep them simple and to the point—uncluttered and with gaps between each line so they are easier to read.
- Break down the instructions—to say tidy the kitchen isn't clear enough, break down each task, such as: put the dirty breakfast bowls in the sink and add washing liquid (1 squirt) add hot and

cold water then wash. And so on.

- Whenever you meet a child or adult with EF difficulties whatever their age, start where they are at, do not over complicate things because they are an adult. Age has nothing to do with ability or expectations.

- Some children will respond to lots of praise whilst others will not, it can for some create too much attention on them and feel too intense, so they will refrain from doing tasks. This can be figured out—whatever their preferences, abide by them—not everyone needs loads of praise whilst others thrive with it.

- Drawing a visual map—of say a rucksack (an example) then either use small photos of what is to go in there for that particular day for school, then the child can use this (with support from a LA (learning assistant) if they have one, or for themselves to ensure they put everything back to take home, including PE kits and iPads, etc.

- Visual maps, instructions can be put in a phone, an exercise book, have alarms set up to aid memory recall—find ways that can positively and discreetly (if necessary) especially if the young person is in high school, help them to remember what to do and when.

- Remember the main goal, throughout this book I have mentioned that everything can take time, years, even to master. When we are children, we go through loads of changes that are an array of hormone rebalances, mental, physical, emotional and sensory developments and not all at the same time. Add to that tiredness, illness, environment, people and places—nothing stays the same and none of this develops in a straight line.

- Children and adults who have EF and sensory challenges do not do things just for attention, they are genuine needs and difficulties however small or obvious things may seem to the outsider looking in.

- Listen to the young person and how they feel, what they are finding difficult and why. Together making plans to problem solve can be more beneficial so that the young person is in control of themselves, which in itself is a great learning tool for self-reliance.

Chapter 20
A Summary

- Having extremely sensitive sensory inputs and outputs whether they are hyper or hypo sensitive can affect a person's ability to learn.
- Intellectual Learning Disability is a stand-alone condition with or without autism and sensory processing differences.
- Early Intervention of intentional observation through the sensory lens is a valid and powerful way of learning a child's behavioural and sensory processing communications.
- Being unwilling or able to take part in any activities or social events can be due to sensory issues that cause the inability to interact, which isn't necessarily the same as not wanting to.
- Reframing environments for your child's individual needs can:

  1. Help them engage with activities if they choose to
  2. Help them to engage with other humans if they choose to
  3. Help them feel confident
  4. Help them feel understood
  5. Help them feel accepted
  6. Help them feel seen
  7. Help them feel loved
  8. Help them feel valued
  9. Help them feel confident
  10. Help them feel positive about themselves

11. Empower them to speak up for themselves in any method of communication they choose
12. Prevent them from harmful masking
13. Prevent them from feeling shame around their sensory needs
14. Aid their learning skills
15. Teach you about your child and their personalities
16. Enhance their chances of a happy life
17. Create a loving relationship between you and your child
18. Give them a joyful life
19. Help them have a positive attitude to life and others
20. Remove anxiety and fear from their daily lives
21. Enables them to learn about themselves, building their self-awareness and ability to self-regulate throughout their lives
22. Ensures they can thrive in any environment rather than survive in one
23. Helps to keep them safe and make them learn to recognise their own needs, likes and dislikes—knowing when to say no and yes when it feels right for them
24. All children develop as they experience the world, autistic children are no different when given the right environment that enables their needs to be met.
25. Behaviours expressed are not always what they seem, some behaviours may look like someone is in distress when in fact they are happy and vice versa.
26. Observing and learning from the autistic child/adult is paramount to positively supporting them in every way.
27. Always treat each individual as such, autism is not a one size fits all, it is a complex and intelligent neurotype.

If you are a parent/carer, ensure your child is treated individually, correcting any stereotype phrases or labelling or assumptions.

Some behaviours and expressive communication are about feeling poorly and in pain, always check that the person is healthy and free of pain, never assume it is a part of their autism or sensory processing until, you are sure.

There isn't a person on this earth who is an expert in autism, whilst there are those who have studied, researched and know a lot of good stuff and will positively support your individual needs, there are those who cannot, be mindful of this. Taking time to find the people/professionals that feel right and fit your child and their needs. Speaking with other autistic people of all ages and identities can and will give you golden knowledge that you can use to help learn about and support your child.

Stereotyping still exists within the autistic realms, moving away from this makes it easier to see that there is much to learn and understand about every human who is autistic. Like any neurotype there is a spectrum of abilities and disabilities. Some autistic people will need more levels of support than others.

Stereotyping labels such as high and low functioning are being strongly discouraged by autistic communities around the world. They usually create stigma and invalid assumptions about a person's needs and abilities which has fundamental impacts that are usually negative.

Most humans are high and low functioning in many areas of life and experiences, this isn't exclusive to the autistic neurotype. We do not use these terms in any other condition as it doesn't give any valuable information about a person—it's too ambiguous so instead, we list levels of support that are needed in a person's life.

Meeting autistic people, whatever their age or support needs, is an opportunity to learn more about the human psyche. We are all complex and incredible, unique and amazing. Acceptance and compassion, listening and supporting are the attributes of a healthy and thriving community, whether that is home, school, workplace or anywhere.

Families need professional minds that can help advocate and empower clients and their children as they navigate through their lifetime, working together is beneficial to all concerned.

I hope this book has enhanced your knowledge with regards to the combination of autism and sensory processing challenges. Although only an introduction to such topics—my intention is that you will feel you have learnt more about your child or client in the reading of it.

Maybe it has given you more questions, or eased your way into parenting and finding different strategies that can support your child in ways you did not know before.

Anyone you meet who is autistic will be experiencing some of the challenges in their sensory processing, now I am hoping you will recognise some of them and be able to offer support and compassion if you see anyone struggling.

Thank you for reading my book, it has given me great pleasure in the creating of it and I am keen to write more for there is much to explore and share.